OVERCOMING DYSLEXIA

Dr Bevé Hornsby is a clinical psychologist, teacher and speech therapist – possibly the only person qualified in all three fields in Britain. She ran the Speech Therapy Clinic in Kingston-upon-Thames from 1969–72, was Head of Remedial Teaching at St Thomas's Hospital, London, from 1970–1, and took over the Dyslexia Clinic at St Bartholomew's Hospital from 1971–81, building it up into a department in its own right, and into the most famous hospital dyslexia clinic in Britain. Dr Hornsby also started the first one-year teacher training courses in the country in 1973.

Dr Hornsby is an Associate Member of the British Psychological Society, and College Adviser on Dyslexia to the College of Speech Therapists. She has published numerous articles in specialist medical and educational journals, and lectures on dyslexia to doctors, nurses, teacher-training colleges and other professionals. She also runs teacher-training courses throughout the world.

Dr Hornsby retired from St Bartholomew's in 1981, and now runs her own centre at 71 Wandsworth Common Westside, London SW18 2ED, Telephone 081 871 2691/1092.

OVERCOMING DYSLEXIA

A straightforward guide for families and teachers

Dr Bevé Hornsby
PhD, MSc, MEd, MCST, ABPsS

Foreword by
Susan Hampshire
and
Angharad Rees

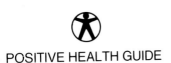

POSITIVE HEALTH GUIDE

To the hundreds of dyslexics I have assessed and taught, who, in turn, have taught me so much.

© Bevé Hornsby, 1984

First published in the United Kingdom in 1984 by
Martin Dunitz Limited, London
Reprinted 1985, 1986

This edition published in 1988 by
Macdonald Optima, a division of
Macdonald & Co. (Publishers) Ltd
Reprinted 1989, 1990, 1991

A member of Maxwell Macmillan Pergamon Publishing Corporation

British Library Cataloguing in Publication Data

Hornsby, Bevé
    Overcoming dyslexia: a straightforward
    guide for families and teachers. — (Positive
    health guide).
    1. Dyslexic children. Remedial education —
    For parents and teachers
    I. Title   II. Series
    371.91′4

    ISBN 0-356-14499-2

Macdonald & Co. (Publishers) Ltd
165 Great Dover St
London
SE1 4YA

Photoset in Garamond

Printed and bound in Singapore

CONTENTS

ACKNOWLEDGEMENTS

I would like to thank those parents and children who have allowed me to use their case histories and written work in this book. To protect their anonymity I have changed their names and minor details of their cases; but in every other respect the case histories are true.

I am grateful to the following colleagues and friends with whom I have been able to share ideas. Miss Maisie Holt, Mrs Marion Welchman and Mrs Sally Childs were among the first to introduce me to the field. Marion Welchman continues to be a staunch and valuable ally and a seemingly unending source of information. I would also like to mention Prof Tim Miles, with whom I had the pleasure and honour of working for a time. Many have had some influence on my thoughts and methods, including Prof Gerald Russell, Dr Trevor Silverstone, Prof Oliver Zangwill, Mrs Sandhya Naidoo, Mrs Helen Arkell, Mrs Wendy Fisher, Dr Harry Chasty, Mr Martin Phillips, Dr George Pavilidis, Dr Margaret Newton, Dr Michael Thomson, Mr Colin Stevenson, Dr Margaret Rawson, Dr Lucia Karnes and a host of others. I would also like to thank my editor, Piers Murray Hill, for his help and encouragement. Finally, I would like to pay particular tribute to my colleagues at the Dyslexia Clinic at St Bartholomew's Hospital, who stood by me so loyally during the difficult and frustrating years when the clinic was being upgraded into a department. They continued to work and teach magnificently under almost impossible conditions. Without their dedication the department would not have come into being.   *Bevé Hornsby, 1984*

The publishers thank the following individuals and organizations:

For permission to reproduce illustrative material: Popperfoto, London (page 11, top); St Bartholomew's Hospital's Department of Medical Illustration, London (page 74); ZEFA, London (pages 13 and 122). The drawing appearing on page 11 (bottom): Copyright reserved. Reproduced by gracious permission of Her Majesty the Queen. The diagrams were drawn by David Gifford.

The cover photograph was kindly modelled by Angharad Rees and Linford Cazenove, and was taken by Dave Brown. The desk and chair are courtesy Wagstaff Office Equipment Group, 36–38 New Oxford Street, London WC1. The location photographs were taken by Dave Brown and modelled by Vivienne, Mark and Alistair Kirkby, and Robert and Thomas Dyton. Location courtesy Vivienne Kirkby. The pine table and chairs were supplied by Pine House, 1 Pembridge Villas, London W2; and the child's desk and stool by Patrick's Toys, Models and Bicycles, 107–111, Lillie Road, London SW6.

The teaching drills on pages 61, 62 (top) and 64 are adapted from *Alpha to Omega* by Bevé Hornsby and Frula Shear, with the kind permission of Heinemann Educational Books Ltd. The key words chart on page 59 is reproduced with the kind permission of Ladybird Publishers, Loughborough, Leicestershire. And the lines printed in the Initial Teaching Alphabet which appear on page 58 are reproduced from *Evaluating the Initial Teaching Alphabet* (1967) by John Downing, with the kind permission of Cassell & Co Ltd, a division of the Macmillan Publishing Co.

FOREWORD

Susan Hampshire

When I was a child people had hardly even heard of dyslexia, let alone knew what the word meant. So when I read Dr Hornsby's book *Overcoming Dyslexia* I was relieved that parents and teachers who do not already know about dyslexia or who need to know more about it, can now gain a better understanding of the problem.

It is a lonely existence to be a child with a disability that no one can see or understand. You exasperate teachers, disappoint parents and, worst of all, know no way of proving that you are not stupid. At school, I used to wait in terror for my teacher to point her finger at me and say, 'Susan, you stand up and read the next two paragraphs.' As I struggled to decipher the words, perspiration would roll down my arms and make little patches on the floor. Yet I was lucky. I went to my mother's school and was protected and encouraged to build up an ability for hard work, patience and determination – qualities I have been grateful for ever since. But I know many dyslexics whose confidence has been badly shattered by fellow classmates at school, and who have never been given the right kind of help.

There is a desperate need for a wider understanding of how dyslexia can be tackled at home, at school and in later life. I think this easy-to-read book meets that need. It is optimistic, full of practical advice and in my opinion no teacher or parent of a dyslexic child should be without it.

Angharad Rees

My son, Linford, who appears with me on the cover of this book, is dyslexic. He is also exceptionally bright, having an IQ of over 130. In his first year at school, Linford made no progress at all with reading and writing. Ignoring his obvious intelligence, his teachers thought that he was slow, told us not to worry and said there was nothing we could do. I am dyslexic myself, so was lucky to be able to recognize the warning signs. I took Linford at the age of six to see Dr Bevé Hornsby, who diagnosed him dyslexic. At his assessment he was unable to recognize any letters of the alphabet. He then began specialist tuition with a teacher trained in Dr Hornsby's methods, which are described in this book.

Linford's transformation was miraculous – he is now nine years old, with a reading age of twelve and a spelling age of eleven. Thanks to early detection and the right kind of help he is doing well at school, works tremendously hard and enjoys life to the full. In short, he has overcome his dyslexia. I can't thank Dr Hornsby and her colleagues enough for saving Linford from a lifetime's struggle with his disability. How wonderful that this book at last makes her wisdom and experience available to all who need them. My hope is that it will help to make success stories like Linford's the rule rather than the exception.

INTRODUCTION

Dear Dr Hornsby,
I am writing to you out of sheer desperation. I have a
son, John, aged eight and a half, who is causing me a
tremendous amount of worry. A few weeks ago his
teacher said that his reading age is only about six. His
writing and spelling are appalling. His IQ has been
checked and is said to be average. I know that he is not
stupid, in fact he is quite bright. He is practically at
the bottom of his class and going backwards.
*   Would you please help me somehow to see if we can*
define his problem and solve it. I would be prepared
to give up my job as a nurse if it was necessary for me
to work constantly with John on any remedial work
that may be necessary, as I know there is something
there somewhere.

This cry from the heart is typical of the many letters I receive regularly from distraught parents. I can well understand their anxiety. In today's society literacy is the key to success at school and, often, to employment. If you have noticed that your child is falling behind in his reading and writing, yet seems bright enough, then naturally you will be worried: might there be something seriously wrong with him? how is he going to cope at school? will this problem have any long-lasting effects on his future life? You may also be concerned that others might think he is stupid, or just plain lazy.

As I shall be explaining throughout this book, dyslexia is most certainly not a sign of low intelligence, nor is it simply the middle-class parents' excuse for their child's backwardness or idleness. It is a common diagnosable condition that is estimated to affect at least one child in ten. A significant proportion of the adult population is dyslexic too – including such well-known successful personalities as Susan Hamphire, Angharad Rees, Beryl Reid, Sarah Miles and British Olympic swimming champion, Duncan Goodhew, to name but a few.

My own interest in dyslexia was aroused in the late 1960s when, as Head of the Speech Therapy Clinic at Kingston-upon-Thames near London, one of my research projects showed that the vast majority of young children with an early speech impediment later developed difficulties with reading. In 1971 I took over as Head of the Dyslexia Clinic at London's St Bartholomew's Hospital. At that time the clinic had only two qualified staff. Such was the demand for skilled help, that by 1981 our team had expanded to twenty specialist teachers, who saw between them over 170 dyslexics a week. While at the clinic I carried out a study on 243 dyslexics into the causes of the condition; and many of the facts and statistical figures appearing in the pages that follow are based on the results of this study and are published here for the first time.

I hope that my book will pass on some of the insights my work has given me into dyslexia, and help dyslexics, their parents and schoolteachers to understand and tackle successfully the problems it can cause. If, by raising public awareness of dyslexia, this book also leads to improved facilities for recognizing and teaching dyslexics, then it will fully have achieved its purpose.

In the first half of the book I show how dyslexia can affect every aspect of a child's life, describe the symptoms, and advise parents and schoolteachers on what practical help they can give. Later on, I explain the diagnostic tests your child might be given, show how successful specialist teaching can be, give tips on how students and adults can cope with their dyslexia, and finally take a look at the latest theories on its causes. But first, of course, we need to know exactly what dyslexia is; and it is with this question that I shall begin.

1. WHAT IS DYSLEXIA?

The word 'dyslexia' comes from the Greek meaning 'difficulty with words or language'. Perhaps the simplest modern definition of dyslexia is that it is difficulty in learning to read and write – particularly in learning to spell correctly and to express your thoughts on paper – which affects those who have had normal schooling and do not show backwardness in other subjects.

This definition is helpful in so far as it describes what every dyslexic has in common. But it does not tell the whole story. Although dyslexia is still widely thought of in terms of so-called 'word blindness', there are many other problems, less well known, that may be associated with the condition. A dyslexic child may have trouble in differentiating between left and right, in learning to tell the time or tie shoe-laces, or in following instructions, for instance, or might confuse spoken sounds – such as /v/, /th/ and /f/ in words like 'live', 'lithe' and 'life'. There are many other possible difficulties, all of which I shall be looking at more closely in Chapter 3.

The fact that dyslexia can show itself in so many ways and can result from different causes (see pages 15–17) has created disagreement among some doctors, psychologists, teachers and educational establishments. You may come across sceptics who say that because the symptoms are so diverse and do not always occur together in the same person, there can be no such single condition as dyslexia. This confusion arises because it is a general umbrella term covering such a wide range of related symptoms. No one would argue that because there are so many varieties of rose – each with its own distinctive colour, shape, size and smell – you therefore cannot call each type of specimen a rose. So it is with dyslexia: one dyslexic child may have a very different set of dyslexic characteristics to another, but will share with all dyslexics the specific difficulty of learning to read, write and spell.

I suspect that many of those who say that dyslexia does not exist have never been closely associated with a dyslexic. I am sure that many parents and teachers would agree that once seen, never forgotten! Despite the non-believers, it is now generally agreed by educationalists and the medical profession that there is such a condition and, as confirmation of this, legislation now exists in several Western countries, including Britain and the United States, that people diagnosed dyslexic must receive adequate treatment.

Is dyslexia related to intelligence?

A more complete picture of dyslexia will emerge as you read through the book, but it is very important to make it clear at the start that dyslexia is not the result of low intelligence, although it is possible for someone of low intelligence also to be dyslexic.

The unfortunate situation which has faced the dyslexic to date is that the ability to read, write and spell is normally equated with brightness. Generally it is true that the link between intelligence and reading ability is very strong; but not in everyone. Most people jump to this conclusion with dyslexics. I have even heard a dyslexic boy's mother say, 'Oh no, my daughter hasn't any problems, she has always been very bright' – implying that her son is not.

The proof that dyslexia is not related to intelligence is that a child with an IQ of 150 – which is extremely high – may still have difficulty in picking up written language skills. In fact, the most distinctive feature of dyslexia is that a child's reading and writing do not measure up to his all-round intellectual ability, at whatever level that might be. Children who are generally backward lag behind in all areas of development – in walking, talking and their ability to solve everyday problems, as well as in reading and writing – whereas the dyslexic is brighter than his written work would suggest. Certainly, most of the dyslexics who were taught at our clinic at St Bartholomew's Hospital in London were of above average intelligence. Although this often made their struggle with reading and writing all the more frustrating, their mental agility nearly always enabled them to respond well to remedial teaching.

Famous dyslexics

The myth that dyslexics are just stupid can most effectively be laid to rest by mentioning some of history's most famous dyslexics – all of them men of exceptional ability and intellect. I hope this will be reassuring if your child has recently been diagnosed.

Albert Einstein (1879–1955), arguably the greatest scientist of all time, is the name we most commonly associate with genius. He did not begin to read until he was nine, but by the age of twelve was a brilliant mathematician and physicist, despite having no gift for languages. He failed his first attempt at entrance to college, and two years after graduation lost two teaching jobs because of his dyslexic difficulties.

Leonardo da Vinci (1452–1519), the remarkable Florentine artist, architect, engineer and scientist, was undoubtedly dyslexic. Examples of his mirror writing can still be seen in his notebooks in the British Museum in London.

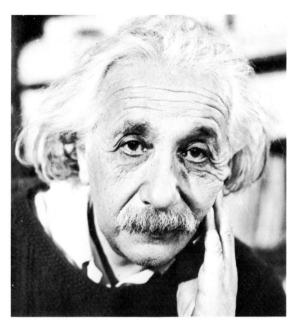

Albert Einstein, whose name we associate with genius, was dyslexic. He did not begin to read until he was nine.

An example of Leonardo da Vinci's mirror writing from his notes on the powers of nature, c 1508.

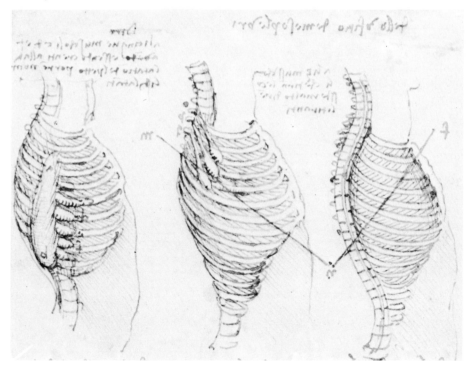

Thomas Alva Edison (1847–1931), the American inventor of the telephone, the microphone, the phonograph and the electric light bulb, among many other things, was thought to be a dunce at school. He could never learn the alphabet or arithmetic tables by heart, and his spelling and grammar remained appalling throughout his life. Here is a sample of his writing at the age of nineteen:

> Dear mother – started store several weeks i have growed coisiderably I dont look much like a Boy now Hows all the fold did you receive a Box of Books Memphis that he promised to send them languages – Your son Al.

Hans Christian Andersen (1805–1875), Danish author of many classic fairy tales, such as *The Ugly Duckling* and *The Snow Queen* was dyslexic. This has only relatively recently been discovered by expert analysis of his handwritten manuscripts.

Auguste Rodin (1840–1917), the famous French sculptor of 'The Thinker', was, according to biographical evidence, the worst pupil in school. His father once said, 'I have an idiot for a son,' and his uncle claimed that he was ineducable. Rodin was eventually given an honorary doctorate by Oxford University when he was sixty-seven years old, although spelling and arithmetic still baffled him.

Woodrow Wilson (1856–1924), President of the United States at the time of the First World War, did not learn his letters until the age of nine and could not read until he was eleven. He was thought to be a dullard at school, but turned out to be a marvellous debater who never needed any notes.

General George Patton (1885–1945), the commander of the American Third Army in western Europe at the end of the Second World War, had a fantastic verbal memory, but could not read well and had to have somebody else to write down his examination answers for him.

Harvey Cushing (1869–1939), the eminent American brain surgeon, studied at Harvard and Yale Universities despite appalling spelling: 'priviledge', 'definate', 'sacarifice', 'pharsical', 'cronicling', and so on. This problem did not prevent his writing several books, including *The Life of Sir William Osler,* which won him the prestigious Pulitzer prize for literature in 1925.

Apart from proving that dyslexics are not lacking in intellect, and showing that dyslexics can often have exceptional skills and insights which are denied to other people, this roll-call of illustrious bad spellers must surely convince even the most hardened doubters that dyslexia exists. How else can you explain why such highly intelligent people were unable to read and write adequately?

Who has dyslexia?

Because experts still disagree about the definition of dyslexia, it has not yet been possible to reach an entirely accurate estimate of the number of people who are dyslexic. Nevertheless I think it is safe to say that recognizable forms and degrees of dyslexia are present in 10 per cent of children in the Western population – and this may well be a conservative estimate. That means that around 1¾ million children in Britain and almost 6 million in North America have difficulty with language. In only 2 per cent of these can dyslexia be considered severe. However, we do have figures which show that in State schools (public schools in the United States) four children out of every class of forty are likely to have difficulty learning to read. Some have early problems which seem to be overcome later and others have continuing trouble. Children whose reading difficulty appears to be

At least one child in ten is likely to be dyslexic to some degree.

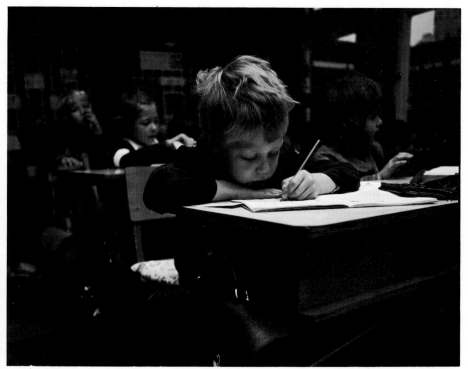

to be overcome do still need to be watched, nevertheless, as they may be the so-called 'hidden dyslexics', whose lack of literacy skills is often not marked enough for their problem to be recognized (see pages 33–8).

You will notice that throughout the book I shall talk about 'he' when referring to a dyslexic. This is because there are more dyslexic boys than girls, the estimates ranging from 4 to 1 up to 7 to 1. This imbalance in numbers is thought to be due to the language area in the brain (see Chapter 9) being usually more mature in girls than boys until puberty in the early teens. This seems to give girls an advantage in picking up linguistic skills during their formative years.

Is dyslexia related to social background?

Although the exact number of dyslexics is not known, there are statistics which show that handicaps of all kinds, including learning disorders like dyslexia, are more common in the densely populated areas of large towns – especially in the less well-off districts – than they are in more affluent sections of society. This is also largely true of isolated country districts, where literacy expectations and quality of schooling may not be as high as in other sectors of the community.

A recent British survey undertaken in 1970 by Prof Michael Rutter and his colleagues on the Isle of Wight – a relatively well-to-do rural district – found that one child in ten had a learning difficulty of one sort or another. In a later study which he conducted in inner London, this figure rose to one in six. Professor Rutter found that 5 per cent of the children in the Isle of Wight study were one year retarded in reading, and 2 per cent were lagging two or more years behind their age and intellectual expectation. In the inner London districts this figure was much higher – as much as 10 per cent.

In poor urban communities there are often a number of factors that make learning difficult: immigrant families' lack of knowledge of the English language, large families inadequately housed, poor diet, environmental pollution, lack of sleep, poor health and possible lack of interest in books and literacy. Add to this the fact that the average number of books in the home is around 1.2 and that many parents do not consider literacy important and so do not, or perhaps cannot, read to their children, it is not surprising that the percentage of dyslexic children in less well-off sectors of society is so high.

Adults

It is not only schoolchildren who have problems with reading and writing. In Britain approximately three million people over school age – over 6 per cent of the total population – have reading ages of less than nine years. A million of these are completely illiterate, being unable to make any practical use whatever of reading and writing in everyday life; while the remaining two-thirds, although able to understand a simple paragraph in a popular newspaper, are not literate enough to cope with even the most basic public information leaflets, such as the Highway Code.

In the United States a recent report by the National Commission of Excellence in Education puts the current figure of illiterate adults at 23 million. It says, for example, that a quarter of the men entering the Navy are unable to read simple safety instructions.

In the developed world, literacy is not only considered to be essential – without it you are handicapped in a society that is run largely through the written word – but is also taken for granted. Until recently it was widely assumed that providing free universal education would guarantee minimal literacy for all children at school. It was not until the early 1970s that it was realized that such a large number of people were leaving school virtually illiterate or semi-literate.

How many of these are actually dyslexic is not known because they have not been systematically investigated. Some are likely to be generally behind in mental skills across the board, while others may have lacked sufficient schooling due perhaps to illness or truancy. These people would not be considered dyslexic according to the definition I gave at the beginning of this chapter. It is reasonable to assume, though, that the vast majority have an adequate verbal knowledge of the language they are expected to read and write, have been adequately taught at school and do not suffer from any physical or mental disability that might make learning difficult, and so are in all probability dyslexic.

The embarrassment and frustration many adults feel who have not learned to read and write can sometimes lead to persistent anxiety or depression that can be bad enough to make them seek help from their doctors. However, dyslexia is no longer something about which adults need to feel ashamed. In my own practice I have met innumerable fathers and some mothers who readily admit to having dyslexic difficulties. These people range in occupation from builders, plumbers, mathematicians, engineers and electricians to members of the British aristocracy, lawyers, architects, doctors, surgeons and teachers. As I shall be showing in Chapter 8, there are many steps the adult can take to overcome the everyday problems caused by his dyslexia.

What causes dyslexia?

As far as we know, there is no single simple cause of all learning disabilities. However, it is now suspected that dyslexics' brain cells may be arranged differently from those who have no difficulty with reading or writing, and that this unusual structure of cells affects to a varying degree the normal functioning of one area or another in the brain. I shall be explaining in Chapter 9 exactly how the dyslexic's brain is affected. It is enough to say here that the root of the problem is thought to be an inefficient connection between the left and right halves of the brain. This might sound alarming stated in such medical terms, but to put it in perspective remember that I am talking about very subtle variations in the arrangement of cells, not the severe brain abnormalities that result in more serious conditions than dyslexia.

Is it inherited?

In a small percentage of cases, learning disabilities in children of normal or superior intelligence are the result of minimal physical damage to the brain, either sustained before or around the time of birth or caused by illness (such as convulsions) or accident later in life. The presence of such damage is difficult to prove as it is so subtle that it does not normally show up on neurological testing. Normally it mostly affects a child's physical coordination. Fortunately, when this is the case, children tend to improve of their own accord, if the lack of dexterity is not too pronounced.

However, evidence is accumulating all the time that a tendency to dyslexia is largely inherited. Certainly, 88 per cent of the children who attended our clinic in London had a positive family history of dyslexia; and often there was a record of more than one child being affected in the same family. In Chapter 4 I shall be giving advice to prospective mothers who have dyslexics in their own or their partner's families as to how they can minimize the risk of their children becoming dyslexic.

Aggravating factors

Poor schooling Constant changes of school, particularly if this also involves drastic changes of teaching methods, may well retard a child's ability to acquire the basic skills in reading, writing and arithmetic.

The extent to which school, teachers and child are compatible are important features in a child's life, especially in his early years. A school that keeps parents at arm's length and does not encourage their participation is unlikely to be a happy one. The attitude of the school's headteacher or principal is also an extremely important factor in the way a school is run. Sympathetic principals tend to attract sympathetic teachers. Children undoubtedly flourish in such a rewarding atmosphere. Conversely, of course, if the school's set-up does not suit a particular child, or teacher and child don't get on with each other, the child may well learn nothing until the situation changes.

Open-plan education, where children do not sit in rows of desks but all do different tasks at little tables dotted about large rooms, may be more fun and suits some children very well. But the dyslexic child who finds it hard to concentrate will be totally lost; he needs a much more structured system of instruction. A change of environment may be all that is needed. Similarly, a child who is not progressing on the modern whole-word method of teaching reading – the so-called 'Look and Say' method – might do better if given more traditional, separate-letter-sound teaching to help him break the code (see Chapter 5).

Poor health The child who is in constant poor health and who never feels really well will have difficulty concentrating on learning at school. Common causes of continuous illness are respiratory tract infections, such as bronchitis, or common colds which lead to stuffy noses, headaches, sore throats and congestion of the middle ear. These in turn may lead to accompanying problems of intermittent hearing loss, or 'glue ears' (see pages 85–6), which is due to congestion, and is bound to affect satisfactory school progress.

The general state of a child's health must always be taken into account when assessing his school achievement. If it is not good, then obviously parents must enlist the continuing help of their family doctor to try to get their child well enough to benefit from the schooling that will help him overcome his dyslexia.

Can dyslexia be cured?

There is as yet no cure for dyslexia, but it is no longer necessary to be distressed if your child is dyslexic, because there are well-tried methods of teaching which greatly improve the condition in the vast majority of cases. As I shall be showing in Chapters 4, 5 and 6, there are innumerable other ways in which dyslexics can be helped by teachers, psychologists, speech therapists, family doctors, and of course by their parents. There is also much that the adolescent and adult dyslexic can do to help themselves (see Chapter 8). But before examining these professional and self-help techniques for coping with dyslexia, I want now to look at many of the common problems that can arise for dyslexics, their parents and teachers, and how they might be avoided.

2. UNDERSTANDING DYSLEXIA

Despite the bright prospects of a normal life for dyslexics offered by today's teaching and other remedial methods, it cannot be denied that in reality dyslexics, their families and teachers do often encounter daunting problems, most of which I believe are based largely on a lack of understanding.

This lack of understanding begins with the child himself who cannot grasp why other children, often less bright than himself, seem to be able to acquire skills in reading, writing, spelling and perhaps arithmetic, which he finds so difficult or even totally incomprehensible. He may react to his failure to keep up in these subjects with temper tantrums, psychosomatic ailments such as headaches or tummy upsets, or by wetting or soiling himself – all of which may alarm his parents and baffle his family doctor. He may also puzzle his teachers by acting up in class, being aggressive towards his classmates or playing truant.

Naturally enough, parents are often puzzled why their child is doing badly at school when he seems bright enough in every other way. They may begin to wonder whether he is indeed as dull or lazy as his teachers seem to suggest, and to become exasperated by his tiresome and seemingly inexplicable behaviour.

Teachers may be totally baffled by the child who does not respond to teaching methods that are successful for most of their other pupils, especially as there is no obvious reason for his lack of progress. It unfortunately sometimes happens that they take refuge in blaming the child or the parents – which only increases the already existing tension and pressures for everyone involved.

Perhaps the best way of seeing how these and other problems arise, what they can lead to and how they can be prevented or overcome is to look at the story of one of the dyslexic boys who was treated at our dyslexia clinic. His case is typical; and there can be few junior or elementary school teachers or families with a dyslexic child who do not find in it echoes of their own experience.

Billy's story

The signs
Eight-year-old Billy was attending a London junior State school. Janet,

his newly appointed English teacher, had not come across anything quite as impossible to decipher as Billy's efforts at homework. It might have been Greek or Chinese for all the sense it made. Not only that, it was such a mess. The letters, if you could call them that, were scribbled down higgledy-piggledy, there was hardly ever a recognizable word among them, and the pages were full of crossings out and smudges.

Janet was not sure whether the smudges were due to Billy being left-handed and therefore brushing over his work as he wrote it, or to his hand being sweaty from the effort of writing (he pressed so hard the marks were visible for pages ahead), or to tears of frustration being wiped off the pages with his grubby fist.

She had noticed that his face always seemed grubby too. He looked untidy as well. His clothes were not dirty but they seemed to be permanently out of place: buttons in the wrong holes, tie askew, shoe-laces undone, socks falling down, shirt hanging out at the back. He looked as though he had been thrown together rather than dressed.

When he had written work to do in class Billy would chew his pen and gaze at his workbook with a look of perplexed incomprehension on his face. And when the class was given reading exercises, his glance would tend to wander longingly to the grass and trees outside the classroom.

He was the only one in his class to have such dire trouble with his reading and spelling. Even his written arithmetic was poor, although he was quick enough when it came to answering mental arithmetic questions. He was certainly not backward, because he was like an adult to talk to and always shone with verbal answers to his teachers' questions.

When Janet had encouraged Billy to do better, his reply had been eloquent: 'I do try, but it never comes out right. I know what I want to say, but I don't know how to write it – the words won't come out of my head into my hand.' This had prompted her to give him a short dictation to see for herself, and it was true. He had not the first idea how to put the words down on paper. His hand did indeed become sweaty and his eyes filled with tears. As soon as she had let him join his friends in the playground, Janet went to talk to the principal to see if he agreed that Billy might in fact be dyslexic.

The delay

When she put the problem to the principal, he took a look at Billy's exercise book, asked his age, and said that because he was still so young, they should wait a while before thinking about sending him to an educational psychologist, since his writing, spelling and reading would probably improve of its own accord as he grew older. Janet was too new at the school to argue with the principal and had to accept this approach as the best solution.

Soon afterwards Janet met Billy's father and mother, who ran a local family grocery business, at a parents' evening, and tried to forestall their badly disguised hostility by suggesting that Billy's lack of progress was shortly to be looked into and some remedies suggested. Reassured a little by her obvious concern for Billy, they nevertheless remained anxious and unconvinced. His mother asked Janet if she thought Billy was just being stupid and lazy, and could really manage to pick up reading and writing if he tried. Janet assured her that she did not think so, but that reading just did not seem to have clicked with him yet. She said that everything possible was being done and that things would come right in time. Billy's father was still concerned that his son's almost total lack of reading and writing ability would seriously hamper his chances at senior school (for children over eleven years old), where Billy was due to go in just over two years' time.

The deterioration

Billy's parents' misgivings were well founded. Six months passed and his written work remained indecipherable and reading virtually non-existent, apart from a few words he had managed to pick up by sight. The principal though, kept his promise and eventually arranged for Billy to see the educational psychologist. But, working in a busy city area of the public education system, it was several months before the psychologist could fit in an appointment with Billy. By then his behaviour had become much worse. He was almost uncontrollable in class, disrupting lessons by fooling about and distracting those who wanted to work. He would neither keep quiet nor sit still and seized every opportunity to pinch or punch other children. At about the same time he began to bribe with chocolate bars and toys other disruptive pupils whom he felt might be on his side. To obtain the items for bribery Billy began to steal from his mother's purse.

A mistaken diagnosis

By the time Billy was first seen by the educational psychologist his bad behaviour at home and at school overshadowed his difficulties with reading and writing, and only cursory consideration was given to his lack of literacy skills. In any case, only his reading was investigated, and as he could read some words and did manage a reading age of seven years (he was now almost ten), the psychologist diagnosed the root cause of his problem to be emotional instability.

Both parents were asked to attend for psychotherapy and Billy was sent to a school for the maladjusted. Unfortunately this was quite the worst place for him to go, as his bad behaviour was not the result of being basically emotionally disturbed, but a reaction to his inability to read and write satisfactorily, despite his initial efforts to do so.

In the wrong environment of the new school, Billy's behaviour deteriorated still further until his parents became really frightened. His aggression was showing itself in many ways but most alarmingly towards his younger sister, who, at the age of four, was already beginning to read well.

Treatment at a dyslexia clinic

As Billy was still learning nothing at the school for maladjusted children, his parents decided to take matters into their own hands and send him back to an ordinary school for normal children. They had recently seen a television documentary about our dyslexia clinic at St Bartholomew's Hospital in London and managed to persuade their family doctor to refer Billy there as he had developed school phobia and had started wetting his bed. The doctor was quite sympathetic to the idea that Billy might be dyslexic, without being totally convinced. Nevertheless, an appointment for assessment was finally made with us when Billy was ten and a half.

We found Billy to be of well above average intelligence, but behind in reading by three years, and four and a half years in spelling. Further tests revealed that he had trouble differentiating between certain sounds in words – in 'big' and 'beg', for instance. He found it difficult to repeat or recite sequences of numbers, months of the year and multiplication tables. And, of course, he also made typically dyslexic mistakes (see the next chapter) in the reading and writing he was able to produce. We had no hesitation in diagnosing Billy dyslexic and offered remedial tutoring at the clinic on a once-a-week basis with homework to be supervised by his parents.

The immediate effect on Billy of this first visit to the clinic was electric. There was a dramatic release of tension when parents and child realized what was wrong and that something concrete and positive was going to be done about it. His new school, too, was relieved, as the poor quality of Billy's reading and spelling could no longer be attributed to bad teaching. Now his problem had been correctly identified the school was able to offer encouragement and active support for Billy's dyslexic therapy programme.

However, the road back to recovery was long, slow and demanding. Although the light had appeared at the end of the tunnel, it took three years of hard work before Billy could read reasonably fluently, and another two before he could spell confidently enough to produce an acceptable essay that did justice to his intellect and knowledge. Although he finally succeeded in passing enough exams to study for a degree at university, he remained a slow reader and an uncertain speller, and will probably carry a chip on his shoulder for the rest of his life.

His success and the problems still facing him were summed up in his class teacher's final school report: 'Billy has done remarkably well and should be proud of himself, as we are. However, he will have to learn not to feel affronted if, because of the lingering traces of his disability, other people don't always appreciate that he is a person of good character and intellect.'

Lessons to be learnt

Billy's story is typical of so many dyslexics, and gives a good overall picture of what dyslexia involves. As I said at the beginning of the previous chapter, it is not just word-blindness; it has far wider implications – educational, psychological, social and medical – affecting every aspect of a person's personality and development.

Fortunately, the future for the dyslexic is improving every day. Public and professional awareness about dyslexia is growing, more expert help is now available than ever before, and, as a result, cases like Billy's are becoming fewer in number. However, mistakes are still made, and many dyslexics do undoubtedly still suffer unnecessary hardship as a result of lack of understanding from parents, teachers and other professionals. What, then, can be learnt from Billy's story?

1. I am certain that had his problem been picked up at an earlier age, his reading and writing could have been further improved to near normal. He would not have lost so much ground and needed so long to catch up. His school and family life would have been much happier and more settled, and his future more assured.
2. Following on from this, it is crucial that parents and teachers are alert to any of the tell-tale signs which might indicate that a child is dyslexic. I shall be describing these in detail in the next chapter.
3. Once parents or teachers suspect dyslexia, they should make every effort to ensure that the child is seen by either an educational psychologist, a school counsellor, a consultant, the family doctor or a professional recommended by the local dyslexia association (see the Appendix for useful addresses). As we have seen in Billy's case, a delay can at worst lead to the wrong diagnosis and therapy, and at best to jeopardizing successful dyslexic treatment.

   A word of warning here. As I have noted before, you may come across a psychologist, counsellor or doctor who does not recognize dyslexia as a problem in itself. However, as you will see throughout this book, the weight of current research shows that it is a specific condition with its own causes, symptoms and treatment. So don't be put off by the sceptics. Keep pushing until you find someone who does recognize dyslexia as a condition and who is willing to help your child on the right road to recovery.
4. Finally, try to make sure that the child receives special dyslexia teaching outside his normal school environment (see Chapter 7), and that his regular teachers complement and support this extra work in class (see Chapter 5).

The all-important first step, then, is to recognize as soon as possible the symptoms that might mean your child is dyslexic. I shall be identifying these in the next chapter.

3. HOW YOU CAN TELL THAT A CHILD COULD BE DYSLEXIC

For the non-specialist, identifying a child as dyslexic is not as straightforward as it might seem. Just as every individual is different, so no two dyslexics are the same. As I explained in Chapter 1, dyslexia can show itself in a confusing variety of ways. The aim of this chapter is to provide a rough guide to many of the different pointers which may show that your child is dyslexic, as well as to some of the signs that are popularly thought to indicate dyslexia, but which in fact generally do not.

In the following section all the pointers except the first are 'maybes'. For although they are very often found in dyslexic children, they are not necessarily present in *all* dyslexics. Also, these pointers might be noticed – usually on their own – in people without reading and writing difficulties.

An ability to fit together complicated toys by the age of two is one of the early signs of intelligence. Later in life, dyslexics' reading and writing skills are below what you would expect from their IQ level.

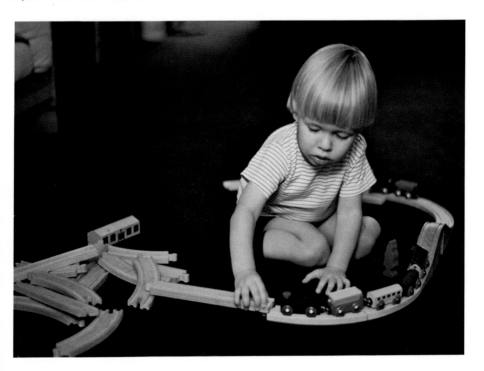

You should also bear in mind that signs of delayed development, such as late walking and talking will also be evident in a child who is generally behind. Only the first of the pointers – lagging behind mental age in reading and writing – is a must. Even then, if there are none of the other accompanying symptoms, there may be other reasons for your child's underachievement. It is only when reading and writing difficulties are linked to one or more of the listed pointers that dyslexia is likely to be diagnosed. The number of symptoms and the length of time over which they occur give an idea of how severe your child's dyslexia might be, which in turn gives a clue to the extent to which it may be able to be overcome with suitable remedial help.

Pointers to dyslexia

He seems much brighter than his reading and written work suggests
Brightness can show itself in a number of ways, other than a child simply being alert to talk to. You may notice that he thinks deeply about the things that go on around him and asks searching and sensible questions. He may show well-developed social awareness, appreciating why certain things, such as taking other children's toys, are done or not done. He may be quick to solve everyday problems. A clever two year old who, for example, having toiled upstairs once or twice carrying only two of his wooden bricks at a time, may decide that this is too laborious and fetch a bag from the kitchen in which to cram as many bricks as possible. He may be exceptionally good at making models from building-block sets, even though he cannot read the instructions. All these signs of intelligence are usually noticable before a child is two years old, but certainly by the time he is five.

Once the dyslexic child arrives at school, his brightness will tend to show more in his verbal skills than his written ones – on average dyslexics are about one to two and a half years behind the reading age you would expect from their IQ (see diagram opposite). However, in the hurly-burly of the classroom it can be difficult for the teacher to differentiate between the bright child who is failing in school achievement because he has a particular disability in acquiring skills in written language and perhaps arithmetic, and the child who is just naughty, lazy, dull or simply not interested in learning. Most children, though, are keen to do well when they start school and you should suspect dyslexia in any who are not progressing, and expert advice should be sought as soon as possible (see page 49). It should be remembered, though, that a five and a half year old cannot be more than six months behind in reading, even if he cannot read at all, as reading tests only start at the five-year level.

The following two lists show typical dyslexic errors in reading and writing. Many of these may, of course, be made by some children in their

24

Reading age prediction chart for non-dyslexics

Using this chart, you can work out a non-dyslexic child's approximate expected reading age from his IQ. For example, an 8-year-old non-dyslexic with an IQ of 105 can be expected to have a reading age of 9. If your child's reading age is below what you would expect from his IQ according to this chart, he may be dyslexic. On average, dyslexics are 1 to 2½ years below their expected reading level. Note, though, that a child of 5½ can only be 6 months behind on a reading or spelling test, as tests do not go below the 5-year level.

Expected reading age of a non-dyslexic, related to his chronological age

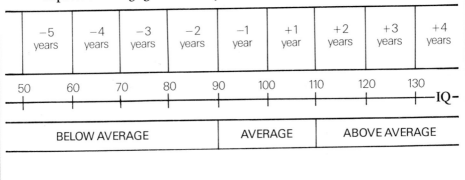

first year at school. Dyslexics, though, will continue to make such mistakes in their second and subsequent school years, once other children have grown out of them.

Typical dyslexic reading mistakes

1. Makes up a story based on the book's illustrations which bears no relation to the text. Bright children often do this rather than admit they are unable to read.
2. Reads very slowly and hesitantly.
3. Follows text with his finger.
4. Constantly loses place, either missing out whole chunks or reading

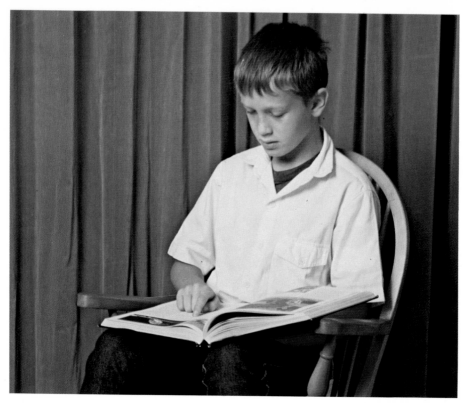

Dyslexics often follow the text with their finger.

the same passage twice.

5. Reads aloud hesitantly, word by word, with little change of intonation – rather like a computerized voice.

6. He may try to sound out the individual elements of words but be unable to synthesize the single sounds into the correct word. For instance, he may sound out b/e/g and then say 'bad', or f/o/g/ and then say 'frog'.

7. Mispronounces words, although they are within the child's vocabulary and can be spoken without any trouble: 'fĭ'nal' for 'fī'nal', 'de'nў' for 'denȳ''.

8. Puts the stress on the wrong syllables, a common mispronunciation being 'phōtōgra'phy' for 'phŏtŏ'graphy'.

9. Reads only in the present tense although the text is in the past. For example, 'The black cat came to my house. She put her kitten by the door,' might be read as: 'The black cat comes to my house. She puts her kitten by the door.'

10. Guesses wildly at words regardless of whether they make sense or not: 'huge' for 'hurt', 'turned' for 'trainer', for example.

11. Reads words backwards: 'on' for 'no', 'saw' for 'was', 'Pam' for 'map', 'God' for 'dog'.
12. Puts letters in the wrong order, reading 'felt' as 'left', 'act' as 'cat', 'reserve' as 'reverse', 'expect' as 'except'.
13. Confuses the short vowels, reading 'beg' as 'bag', 'lid' as 'led'.
14. Misreads initial consonants, either reversing them ('buck' for 'duck'), inverting them ('put' for 'but') or using ones that are visually similar ('how' for 'now').
15. Puts syllables in the wrong order, reading 'animal' as 'aminal', 'hospital' as 'hopsital', 'enemy' as 'emeny'. Or does the same with words: 'Is she' for 'She is'.
16. Foreshortens words: 'rember' for 'remember', 'sunly' for 'suddenly', 'spit' for 'splint'.
17. Misreads words of similar visual appearance regardless of meaning, such as 'help' for 'held', 'disappear' for 'despair', 'though' for 'through', 'house' for 'horse', 'led' for 'let', 'steel' for 'steed'.
18. Substitutes another word of similar meaning, for example: 'go' for 'journey', 'Sunday' for 'Saturday', 'gave' for 'got', 'tree' for 'garden'.
19. Misreads little words, such as 'a' for 'and', 'the' for 'a', 'from' for 'for', 'then' for 'there', 'were' for 'with'.
20. Omits or reads twice little words like 'the', 'and', 'but', 'in'.
21. Adds little words which do not appear in the text.
22. Ignores punctuation, thus often confusing the sense of the text.
23. Omits prefixes, particularly 'un', thus reading 'unhappy' as 'happy', 'unfastening' as 'fastening'.
24. Omits suffixes such as 's', 'ed', 'ing', 'ly' or 'ness'.
25. Adds affixes, reading 'I returned round' for 'I turned round'.

A striking example of how some dyslexics guess wildly at words, regardless of whether they make sense or not, is eleven-year-old Sarah's effort at one of the reading tests regularly given at our clinic. An extract from the test is as follows:

Now the children were discussing their new play. 'We need a brave person for the mountain rescue,' explained a boy. Each puppet tried to appear like the required hero. Then cheers greeted the boy's choice. On the stage was raised the shy but happy Swiss puppet.

Sarah's reading of this passage ran thus:

How the children were designing their new play. 'We need a brave man of the mount chishime,' ixslating a boy. Each puppy tried to apprat the real heeyou. The chance great the boy's chorus. On to the stage was realized the scene but happy Swizz puppy.

Typical dyslexic spelling mistakes

1. Writes letters in the wrong order: 'Simon' spelt 'Siomn', 'time' spelt 'tiem', 'child' spelt 'chidl'.
2. Mirror writes words: 'nomiƐ' for 'Simon'.
3. Reverses letters, writing 'b' as 'd', 'p' as 'q'.
4. Inverts letters, writing 'n' as 'u', 'm' as 'w', 'd' as 'q', 'p' as 'b', 'f' as 't'.
5. Mirror writes letters and perhaps numbers: 'γ' for 'y', '⊦' for '4'.
6. Spells words as they sound: 'busy' as 'bizzy', 'sight' as 'site'.
7. Uses bizarre spellings like: 'last' spelt 'lenaka', 'about' spelt 'chehat', 'may' spelt 'mook', 'did' spelt 'don' or 'to' spelt 'anianiwe'. These words bear little, if any, relation to the sounds in the words.
8. Omits letters: 'limp' spelt as 'lip', 'went' as 'wet' or 'string' as 'sing'.
9. Adds letters: 'went' spelt 'whent', 'what' spelt 'whant', 'would' spelt 'woulde'.
10. Cannot write the appropriate letter when given the sound.
11. Cannot write letters even when they are dictated by name.
12. Cannot pick out letters from a display when the name is called out.
13. Cannot match up the same letters when asked to.

Punctuation may remain an almost totally closed door. The dyslexic is lucky if he manages a capital letter at the beginning of a sentence or a full stop at the end. He may well know about question marks, exclamation marks, speech marks and capitals for proper nouns, but seldom succeeds in using them.

He may have difficulty with mathematics
The language of mathematics is often poorly understood by the dyslexic up until the age of twelve – and even beyond. He may not grasp that the words 'difference', 'reduction' and 'minus' all suggest 'subtraction'. Similarly, he may understand the term 'adding', yet be thrown if asked to 'find the total'. He may also be confused by similar-looking mathematical signs: $+$ and $\times$; $-$, $\div$ and $=$; $<$ (less than) and $>$ (greater than); and so on. Around 60 per cent of dyslexics have difficulty with basic mathematics, although this is often overcome when they are introduced to more intuitive mathematics, and they are often good at geometry.

There may be a family history of late reading or poor spelling
Eighty-five per cent of dyslexics have close members of the family who had, or still have, similar problems with reading and spelling. If a dyslexic has significant difficulty with mathematics, this is usually inherited as well.

He may have directional confusion
This may take a number of forms, from being uncertain of which is left

and right to being unable to read a map accurately. A child should know his own left and right by the age of five, and be able to distinguish between someone else's by the age of seven. Directional confusion affects other concepts such as up and down, top and bottom, compass directions, keeping your place when playing games, being able to hold a hockey stick in the right position to pass to the right or the left, being able to copy the gym teacher's movements when he is facing you, and so on. As many as eight out of ten severely dyslexic children have directional confusion. The percentage is lower for those with a mild condition.

Directional confusion may be the reason for so-called mirror writing and reversing of letters, whole words or numbers. If is often considered to be at the heart of the dyslexic's problems with basic arithmetic, especially where subtraction, multiplication and division are concerned. It probably also explains a lot of the difficulties dyslexics have when getting dressed. Some children dislike activities that need a change of clothes, particularly if they also involve finding a changing room, which may require the child to remember, not only the way, but also the number of the room (whether it is '14' or '41'). Many dyslexic children have been put off swimming for this reason.

Some dyslexics, when learning to play the piano, have more difficulty than most other children in mastering the opposing direction of the movements of the two hands.

He may have been late learning to tell the time or tie his shoe-laces
Most children can tie their own shoe-laces when they start school at five, and are beginning to master the intricacies of telling the time by the age of six. Over 90 per cent of dyslexics are later than average in developing these skills, and around half do not pick them up until the age of ten or later, and even then are not 100 per cent successful. Telling the time is closely related to language skills, and tying shoe-laces, to a good sense of direction – both of which have already been mentioned as pointers to dyslexia.

He may find it difficult to put things in the right order
A number of everyday activities depend on our ability to get things in the correct order. Most dyslexics have trouble remembering the order of the alphabet and numbers, the months of the year, the seasons and the events in the day. Younger children – five- and six-year-olds – also find it hard to sequence the days of the week.

Dyslexic children may have difficulty following verbal instructions if more than one are given at once, particularly if the instructions are fairly complicated or include directions. For example, your child may find it impossible to carry out a request like: 'Go upstairs and fetch your red sock with a hole in so that I can mend it – it is in the top right-hand drawer of the chest of drawers beside the back window.' And he may even be confused by a simple instruction like: 'Go and play outside, but put on your shoes and shut the door after you.' It is much better to break it up into manageable chunks.

Child: 'May I go out and play?'
Adult: 'Yes, but put on your shoes.'
When the shoes are on, continue slowly and very clearly:
'Off you go, but shut the door.'

Nearly all dyslexics have trouble putting written symbols in order – that is, arbitrarily chosen signs such as letters, numbers, shorthand, musical notation, and so forth, that indicate something abstract. Certainly, there can be few dyslexics who have not misordered letters in words and numbers in their sums.

However, most are as good as the next child – if not better – at more practical, less abstract sequences of shapes, lights and non-verbal sounds, as in the popular electronic game Simon. In this the players have to press buttons to repeat an ever-increasing number of sequences of coloured lights, each colour being accompanied by a particular tone or sound. Many of my dyslexic pupils have been expert Simon players, and seem to have no trouble at all with home computers (see pages 119–120).

He may have poor or excellent spatial ability

Dyslexics are generally either very good or very bad at playing or working with two- or three-dimensional shapes. Fortunately, more dyslexics have natural talent in this area than do not.

Poor ability   If by the age of three a child cannot draw a circle or make a reasonable attempt at colouring in pictures and cutting out shapes with scissors, then it is likely that his spatial ability will never be well developed. Other early warning signs may be that he does not like playing with even the simplest jigsaws, shape-sorting toys or building blocks.

When he starts school he will probably find learning to write is especially difficult, and have trouble grasping concepts such as bigger/smaller, longer/shorter, more/less, and so on. For instance, a schoolchild with normal spatial ability should be able to understand by the age of seven that there are the same number of dots in each line when shown two lines of five dots each, one spread out, the other bunched up. Dyslexics of the same age and older may continue to think that there are more dots in the longer line (see opposite).

Excellent ability   Dyslexics who show promise in this area as young children are likely to be extremely good at geometry when they grow older. And by the same token they are often exceptional at chess, card games and computer games. Many of my pupils have become successful scientists and engineers – both professions that require good spatial ability.

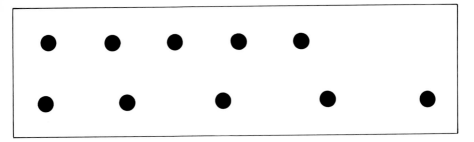

Seven-year-old, and older, dyslexics with poor spatial ability may think there are more dots in the longer line.

He may have trouble putting names to things and people

Many of us cannot put names to faces we know (this tends to happen more often as we get older) but most people can name familiar objects without much difficulty. Around 30 per cent of dyslexics, though, can describe a person or object, while the name eludes them. A boy might know all about the European who discovered the New World, but be unable to recall that his name was Christopher Columbus.

In one of the intelligence tests we use for diagnosing dyslexia, we show a child a comb with some of its teeth missing and ask what is missing. Often the child will point to the teeth that remain and say 'Some of those', failing to find the name for them. Dyslexics' conversation is often peppered with phrases like 'What do you call it?', 'You know what I mean', 'Thinga-mibobs', and so on.

In bright, imaginative children this particular problem can lead to wild fantasies which may puzzle their parents and teachers. I well remember one nine-year-old pupil of mine who, refusing to be put off when he could not recall the name of the person who wrote *Romeo and Juliet*, insisted first that it was the famous English children's author, Enid Blyton, and then, when he guessed that this was incorrect, that the playwright was God!

He may be left-handed or have been late deciding which hand to use

Around 4 per cent of the total population are left-handed, whereas a considerably higher proportion of dyslexics – about a quarter – show a preference for using their left hand, if not actually for writing, maybe for other tasks such as eating, playing two-handed games or using tools.

A child normally begins to show a preference for one hand or the other by the age of one, but should certainly have established a preference by five. Over 70 per cent of dyslexics, whether eventually right- or left-handed, are late deciding which hand to use.

There may be left-handedness or ambidexterity in the family

Nearly 90 per cent of dyslexics have close family who are left-handed or ambidextrous, even when the dyslexic himself is right-handed. Close family would include brothers and sisters, parents, uncles and aunts, grandparents and possibly first cousins. Where there is a family history of dyslexia, but *not* of left-handedness, I have found the dyslexic's condition is not so severe nor so difficult to treat.

He may have been a late or poor talker, and may still have immature speech

Sixty per cent of dyslexics were late talkers. Again, parents will be the first to notice if a child is late starting to talk and whether his speech is clear when it does begin to emerge.

A child should understand simple words and commands from nine months old and may do so earlier. He should be using his first words with meaning at around a year, have a vocabulary of up to 200 words at two, and be using simple two-word phrases – such as 'eat egg' – by then. By three he should have a vocabulary of up to 900 words and be using full sentences with no words omitted. He may still mix up his consonants – 'miggle' for 'middle', for example – but his speech should be comprehensible to strangers. By four, talking should be in full flood with endless questions about everything under the sun, although he may still make grammatical errors such as 'me want it,' or 'I runned away.' By five, he should have acquired basic language, and only the complexity of usage and vocabulary will improve with the years.

If a child still has a speech defect, however mild, or uses immature grammatical structure in his sentences when he starts school at five, this should alert parents and teachers to probable future problems with reading and spelling. In addition to mispronunciations, muddled syllables ('hopsital', 'emeny'), spoonerisms ('par cark' for 'car park', and 'shoving leopard' for 'loving shepherd') and swopping round of words ('take over' for 'overtake') there are other immaturities of grammatical usage – 'Me and Poppa went for a walk,' instead of 'Poppa and I went for a walk,' for instance – which can persist until the teens or even occasionally into adulthood. The dyslexic also often lacks understanding of simile, metaphor and the verbal pun – in other words, of the more abstract and sophisticated uses of language.

Of course, there are always exceptions to every rule, and some dyslexics as well as non-dyslexic children start talking very late in complete sentences without apparently having gone through all the usual stages of language development described above.

He may have been a late walker and not be well coordinated

Twenty per cent of dyslexics were late walkers. Children usually take their first uncertain steps around twelve to fifteen months of age and are walking well enough by eighteen months to no longer have to think about it – the activity has become automatic. If a child is not walking by eighteen months or later there may be cause for concern. Of course, there are a number of possible reasons for a child learning to walk late, including poor health and lack of experience, due, perhaps, to being cooped up in a cot or crib for too much of the time. These may have no effect on the future learning capabilities of that child.

Dyslexics are popularly thought of as being clumsy and accident prone, but while some dyslexic children are not well coordinated, many do brilliantly at sports. Clumsiness is not nearly such a significant early pointer as late talking or even late walking. However, it is as well to bear it in mind. If your child is badly coordinated, sports like trampolining, judo and swimming can help to build up his confidence in his own physical abilities, and usually results in an overall improvement in coordination.

Finding the 'hidden' dyslexic

The more severe a dyslexic's condition and the more signs and symptoms he shows the easier it is for parents and teachers to notice. It is often the borderline children – the 'hidden' dyslexics – who cause the most concern because they are the ones who slip through the net. It is only when they are approaching examinations that their teachers begin to wonder why their written work does not match up to earlier promise. If a child can read, however slowly, hesitantly and inaccurately, it is often assumed that he cannot be dyslexic. This is where the first big mistake may be made. Often teachers and parents do not seem to realize that children may be learning a reading scheme by heart, thus giving the impression of being able to read.

Children's spelling may not always be systematically checked, yet this is one of the easiest things to do, as spelling tests can be given as a class activity or as a game at home. At school the possibility of copying from one another has to be taken into account, of course, but if the test is accompanied by five minutes of free composition without any help from the teacher (see examples on pages 35–7), inadequacies are bound to come to light in even the borderline dyslexic's work. These children should then be further checked individually.

At school it is more difficult to give a reading test to a group, as it must either involve filling in a suitable word which has been left out of a sentence or choosing a suitable word to complete a sentence from a choice of five. This alternative-choice method is not a very reliable guide to reading ability as a child has a 20 per cent chance of being right if he chooses a word at random. Reading tests are best given individually, but this is time-consuming and so may not always be possible at school.

Parents, of course, have more opportunity to hear their children read than do teachers. In my experience many parents have felt that something was wrong with their child's reading or writing even before he started school. If your own suspicions are confirmed within your child's first year at school, then you should not hesitate to raise the matter with his teacher. You run the risk of being labelled 'fussy parents', but for the sake of your child's future it is worth it.

There is another reason why some children's dyslexia is missed until it is too late to prevent it damaging their career. An intelligent child may well learn to cover up his problem by skilful evasion or by getting help with his homework. So it is that the gulf between what he obviously knows and what he can express on paper may not show itself until he takes important exams. The answer lies in schools holding their own written examinations and tests on a regular basis so that dyslexic symptoms come to light quite early on in a child's career and the problem can be looked into before it gets out of hand. But bear in mind that many children who cannot pass examinations are not dyslexic. Specialist investigation will show whether this is the case or whether a first-class brain is being wasted for want of the right kind of remedial help.

Pointers to the 'hidden' dyslexic
Teachers and parents should be on the alert for any of the following difficulties, as any one of them could be a sign that a child is mildly dyslexic.

Poor concentration   The child who does not appear to pay attention to what is going on in class or to listen to what his parents are saying may not be doing so from choice. It may not be a question of 'must pay more attention', but more of 'cannot pay more attention', because a young dyslexic's nervous system is not yet able to cut out unwanted distractions to allow him to concentrate only on what his teacher or parents are saying.

Bad at copying from the board   A child who is unable to copy accurately from the board may not be suffering from poor eyesight, but may lack the ability to retain in mind what he is looking at from a distance long enough to be able to transfer it to paper. And when he looks at the board again for further information he may be unable to find his place. All this will make him a very slow copier, and often the board will be wiped clean before he is even half finished.

Since most teachers write young children's homework on the board or give it to them verbally to write down, the child whose reading and writing skills are not as good as they should be will most probably take home incomprehensible or incomplete instructions. His poor homework performance, therefore, may not mean that he is lazy, but that he is mildly dyslexic.

Badly organized   A child who can never get himself ready to leave for school on time in the mornings, who is always late for lessons because he

Non-dyslexic girl

I live in a small village on the outskirts of West Berlin. I would like to explain the political situation of Berlin both East and West. Many people become confused by this unusual situation and I am going to attempt to clarify it. The Four Power Agreement was signed by the four military powers who administer Berlin. These powers are the British, French, American and Russian military

The city of Berlin is divided by the wall into two parts, East and West Berlin. The Russians control East Berlin and West Berlin is again divided into three sectors.

Five minutes' free writing by a twelve-year-old non-dyslexic girl. The handwriting is well formed with an even slope. The sentences are well constructed and mature, and describe clearly what the writer wants to convey. There are no spelling mistakes. Compare this with the two dyslexic examples overleaf.

Borderline dyslexic girl

It was a cold morning I was out walking ~~fes~~ toby and Lucy my two dogs when a horse came galloping up the Bridle-Path walk down to me it stop and I to See if there was a rider, the horse had tack on. By the time I reached the bottom they was no sighn of any body we walk on the hors Suddenly stopped and would not go forward I Said to him, "Come on It's all right there no one here" The two dogs had gone off to Play Some game. I mounted this horse and we walk forward he did not like It Suddenly he reared up and this man wath a maock Pulled me off this horse.

Five minutes' free writing by a borderline dyslexic girl approaching her thirteenth birthday. Her handwriting is immature and does not keep to a straight line. The sentences are disjointed and do not flow. She does not use capitals for proper names nor, sometimes, for the pronoun 'I'. She leaves out suffixes ('ed') and small words ('is'), and muddles up 'they' and 'there'. Her grammar and punctuation are poor and she has misspelt 'sign' as 'sighn' in line 9, and 'mask' as 'masck' in line 19.

36

Severely dyslexic boy

Translation 'One night there was a fire in a building one man was very injured he was rushed to hospital and three days he died from internal injuries the building was declared unsafe, and the firemen went back to the station.'

Five minutes' free writing by a 14½-year-old severely dyslexic boy of average intelligence. He had a reading age of 7 years, 8 months, and a spelling age of 6 years, 10 months. His writing contains many typically dyslexic mistakes: no punctuation; no capitals (except where used incorrectly); letters swopped round and wrongly ordered—'saw' for 'was', 'for' for 'from'; suffixes and prepositions left out; incorrect tenses; letters positioned wrongly; bizarre spelling; and immature sentence structure.

cannot find his way from classroom to classroom, or who never seems to have the right books and equipment for each lesson, may not be just an absent-minded daydreamer, but have genuine dyslexic difficulties. Not only might he find it hard to remember the correct sequence of the day's events, but he may also mix up the directions in which he is meant to go and be unable to make sense of the school timetable.

Rejection by his age group The child who does not seem to have many friends or is the butt of teasing and being made fun of may be in this position because he is different in ways that are not obvious to his parents or teachers. It is easy to understand that a child who is physically different, in being very fat, very thin, very tall, very small, flat-footed, greasy haired or knock-kneed could be the object of ridicule, as children are often very unkind to one another. But if he is none of these things and still provokes an unfriendly reponse from his fellows, his dyslexic behaviour may be the cause. His peers may think him odd for not being able to do up his shoe-laces or tell the time, for instance, or for spoiling games by not knowing his left from his right.

Lack of self-control Some dyslexic children are naturally resilient and self-assured enough to cope with teasing and the other frustrations of their condition either by laughing at themselves or by ignoring their schoolmates' jibes. Others, though, like Billy in the previous chapter, become sulky, argumentative, aggressive and difficult for parents or teachers to handle.

This kind of behaviour, like all the other possible pointers to the 'hidden' dyslexic I have mentioned, can be unrelated to dyslexia. Nevertheless, they so often are linked that once they have been noticed, arrangements should be made to have the child's reading and writing ability assessed. If dyslexia is diagnosed and treated early enough, the child should be able to overcome many of the problems that alerted his parents or teachers to his condition in the first place.

Mistaken pointers

There are several common childhood problems that are popularly but wrongly assumed to be signs of dyslexia. Every dyslexic's family will know how upsetting it can be for a child to be teased or accused of being backward, lazy or emotionally disturbed, when they and he feel sure that he is none of these things. It is important that these myths are exposed not only so parents can reassure their children and advise them how to cope with such taunts, but also because they create confusion and concern for parents and teachers too. And of course it is vital that children who really do have any of the following problems are given help that is specifi-cally directed at solving these, rather than therapy for dyslexia.

Generally backward
As I have pointed out in Chapter 1, the child who is mentally backward will be behind in developing all skills, from toilet training and social behaviour to reading, spelling, arithmetic and all other school subjects.

There is a diagram on page 25 which shows how you can predict a non-dyslexic child's reading age from his IQ. A rough guide is that there is one year's difference in expected reading age for every 10 points of IQ. In other words, a child with an IQ of 90 (lowest limit of the Average range) should be reading to one year below his actual age; and another with an IQ of 80, two years below. But because he will also be one or two years behind in all subjects across the board relative to his IQ level, he is not dyslexic. His problem is not a specific difficulty with learning to read and write. A child with an IQ of less than 50 will probably have great difficulty learning to read on any but the most basic level.

Emotionally disturbed

Emotional disturbances can broadly be categorized in two distinct groups: those that arise from within the child for no obvious reason, and those that are caused by an external event, such as the arrival of a new baby.

The first type will almost certainly interfere with a child's intellectual development, since he becomes so turned in on himself that he cannot respond positively to experiences and stimulation at school or at home.

The second type, triggered by an upsetting domestic crisis, may temporarily prevent progress at school. Once the problem has passed, though, the child will return to his usual self, his sleep reverting to normal and his learning resuming where it left off.

The thing to remember about emotional disturbances, of whatever kind, is that, like backwardness, they seldom hinder just one aspect of learning, such as reading and writing, but affect every facet of school life. The child may be unable to learn anything at all while he is upset. A visit to your family doctor, or perhaps a psychiatrist, is the right course of action.

Hyperactive

Hyperactivity is a neurological condition. A genuinely hyperactive child is always restless, never sits still for a moment, fidgets incessantly, demands constant attention and sleeps poorly. Although this nervy behaviour is certainly a barrier to learning, it should not specifically prevent a child from learning to read and write. As few as one dyslexic in a hundred is genuinely hyperactive, so hyperactivity is not a useful pointer to dyslexia. Dyslexics, as we have seen, may have difficulty concentrating and often seem bored and fidgety in class. This is due not to hyperactivity but to losing interest in impossible tasks of reading and writing.

Lazy and disinterested

This is really more a general matter of personality than a pointer to any particular condition. Some children are by nature much more academically inclined than others, while some prefer practical activities, sports and having fun. A lucky few seem able to combine all of these. There are, for sure, some dyslexics who seem lazy at school – often because their difficulties make them bored with written work. But so are millions of other children. There is no evidence to show that laziness or lack of interest are any more reliable as pointers to dyslexia than having blue eyes.

Teachers and parents should never automatically assume that a child who shows more enthusiasm for practical rather than written subjects, and who has poor results in English is dyslexic. He might simply not be interested in English as a subject. If so, he will learn to read and write in time without specialist help, but may continue to hate English.

Lack of academic interest may not be so noticeable during a child's early years at school, but can usually be detected as examinations approach. It should be reassuring to know that, as I have already mentioned, many children who fail exams are not dyslexic – another mistaken pointer!

Should dyslexics be identified?

The task of actually diagnosing whether your child's difficulties are due to dyslexia or to other causes is not simple. It is a job that should really be left to the professionals, who have the time, expertise and equipment to perform the very careful assessments that are necessary (see Chapter 6).

This chapter is not designed to be used for do-it-yourself diagnosis, but rather to help you get a better idea of what dyslexia involves, and to alert you to the signs that should prompt the first steps towards having your child's problem properly identified.

Many parents, though, once they suspect that their child is dyslexic, are concerned at the prospect of his being given an official label that proclaims his disability for all the world to see. You may be worried about your child being made to feel 'different', or about the unwarranted social stigma that some people attach to dyslexia, mistakenly believing it to be a type of mental deficiency. However, the benefits of having your child's dyslexia identified far outweigh these possible disadvantages, and I would urge you, for the following reasons, not to allow your anxieties to hold you back.

1. If your child's problem is not identified, there is the risk of his being placed in a remedial class for backward children. This will not only destroy a bright child's self-confidence but starve him of the intellectual stimulation he so badly needs.

2. In many developed countries, including Britain and the United States (but not, unfortunately, Australia or New Zealand), once a child is diagnosed dyslexic, he has a legal right to receive adequate and proper remedial help.

3. Dyslexic children in Britain, North America and Australia may be able to get allowances made for them in examinations (see Chapter 8.)

4. Public awareness and interest in dyslexia has increased enormously over the last few years. There is much less misunderstanding than there used to be and I have found that people generally show a much more sympathetic and helpful attitude towards dyslexics.

5. Finally, and most important of all, it is worth repeating that in my experience identification of the problem has proved, in the overwhelming majority of cases, to be the turning point on the road to recovery. Once the child, his parents and teachers realize that he is not stupid or lazy, a great burden is lifted, tensions are defused and all concerned can work positively towards overcoming his dyslexia and making his home and school life more normal and relaxed. Exactly what practical help parents and teachers can give I shall be describing in the next two chapters.

4. HOW CAN PARENTS HELP?

You will remember from Chapter 1 that around nine dyslexics out of every ten have close family with reading and writing difficulties – strong evidence that a tendency to dyslexia, like athleticism and manual dexterity, is largely inherited. If you know there is dyslexia in your family and you have, or are planning to have children, then there is a whole range of preventive measures you can take – from the time of conception onwards – to lessen the severity of the problem, should your child in fact turn out to be dyslexic. If he doesn't, your efforts will not have been wasted, as they will help him to develop quickly and achieve his full potential.

The remaining 10 per cent of dyslexics, do not inherit their disability. They acquire it, as we have seen, as a result of illness or accident, usually before, or soon after birth. However, parents may be alerted by late talking, among other things, as early as the first year of their child's life that he may have dyslexic problems later on. Again, early help, from babyhood onwards, can make all the difference between dyslexia being a mild hindrance or a major stumbling block later in life.

Obviously, for his first five years a child relies totally on his parents for the right help to minimize the severity of his dyslexia. As soon as he starts formal schooling, responsibility for assisting him cope with his problem begins to shift more onto his teachers, but parents still undoubtedly have a crucial supporting role to play. A specialist dyslexia teacher, too, should feature prominently in his education if at all possible. I shall be showing how schoolteachers can get the best from their dyslexic pupils in the next chapter, and looking in detail at the work of dyslexia specialists and its results in Chapter 7. In this chapter I want to give parents an idea of what practical steps they can take to help their child both before and after he starts school.

How you can help during pregnancy

Mothers or prospective mothers who are aware that there might be a possibility of their child being dyslexic should pay particular attention to their health during pregnancy, as indeed should all mothers.

There is increasing medical evidence that the time between conception and birth may be more important for subsequent growth and development of the child than we realize. During this prenatal period the human foetus

41

is more susceptible to his environment than he may ever be again in his life. What happens to him during these nine months can help to sustain normal development or hinder him from ever achieving his full genetic potential. Several factors over which the mother has some control play a part in creating the baby's environment in the womb, the most important being the mother's general state of health, how tired she becomes each day and the quality of her diet. In addition, smoking, drinking alcohol to excess, and taking certain drugs – especially stimulants, tranquillizers and diuretics, or fluid-reducing pills – can all have detrimental effects on the foetus's development.

It is possible that a poor start before birth may either lead to learning disorders like dyslexia or make them worse in a child who is already genetically destined to inherit them. So if you are pregnant, it makes sense to check with your family doctor or obstetrician exactly how you can help your baby get the best possible start in life – especially if dyslexia runs in your family.

How you can help from birth to school age

Whether you are worried that your child may have inherited dyslexia, or that because he is late in reaching certain stages of development, such as walking and talking, he might be behind in learning to read and write when he gets older, there is plenty you can do to help him make the most of his innate abilities.

It might seem surprising that assisting your child to progress in areas other than reading and writing can play a part in combatting dyslexia, but when a child shows improvement in one aspect of his development, he will do better in others too.

Before getting down to practicalities, there is one golden rule that should govern every parent's approach to dyslexia. It is important that you should not become overanxious about your child's progress, nor communicate any anxiety to him. And above all, do not make him feel under pressure to do well or improve. Constant comparison with your other children or friends' children can be soul-destroying for all concerned. It goes without saying that he must be loved and felt wanted for what he is and how he is. Nevertheless, it is possible to help him, to provide practical encouragement and expand his experience and intellectual growth without in any way pressurizing him to succeed in tasks for which he is not yet ready or which he finds particularly difficult or even impossible.

Walking
Help your baby first to stand, and then to walk at his own pace rather than trying to force progress. At around six months babies enjoy being held standing on your lap, and there's no harm in doing this as long as

your baby shows enthusiasm for it. By eleven months he may be able to pull himself up to stand, grasping you or an item of furniture for support. Give him plenty of scope to do this, but make sure that precarious and harmful objects are kept well out of reach – painful accidents can make him lose confidence. About four weeks later he may start to shuffle cautiously around, holding onto solid objects for support. Do not try to make him walk holding your hands – he probably won't like the feeling, and the more tumbles and accidents he has, the less he will be interested in learning to walk unaided.

Once he has reached this stage, it should not be long before he takes a few steps unsupported. Don't hurry him, but give him the chance to do well by positioning supporting furniture sensibly, by not encouraging him to walk on slippery surfaces and by letting him play barefoot on hard surfaces – socks act like ice-skates at this age! There is no need to use mechanical gadgets like baby-bouncers to strengthen his leg muscles. He will get the knack of walking just as quickly without them.

Talking

Picking up talking skills is the most important part of the dyslexic child's early development and you cannot give too much encouragement in the way of talking to your baby and communicating with him by means of gestures and facial expressions. He will automatically take in what he can and disregard the rest until he is mature enough to make sense of it. If you don't give your child enough of this sort of stimulation his intellectual progress – and especially his later verbal ability – is bound to suffer.

You should begin talking to your baby from the day he is born. Babies can hear at birth and show a marked interest in the sound of a human voice from very early on. In the first weeks it is the tone of voice that matters, rather than what you actually say. Some mothers feel foolish talking to their babies, knowing that they can't understand, and may be at a loss for words. The thing to do is give a running commentary on whatever you are doing with him at the time. Tell him what you are doing as you get him dressed, for instance, or as you are bathing him. Don't make it a one-sided monologue, though, listen to his noises too and respond to them. He wants a chat, not a lecture!

The same basic technique should be used as your baby grows into a toddler. You should explain simply all the time to your child what you are doing with or to him. For example, as you are getting him ready in the morning, say 'Socks – on feet – this foot – that foot – toes in – now shoes – this foot – that foot', and so on. The more repetitions you can manage, the better, as a child who is just beginning to talk has to hear a word some 500 times before it has a chance of becoming part of his vocabulary.

To speed up comprehension, accompany your words with actions whenever you can. For instance, say 'hot', using the appropriate gestures of pulling your hand quickly away and making a face to show that it hurts.

If your child is clearly having difficulty understanding speech by the age of fifteen to eighteen months, it is vital that you talk very slowly and clearly to him, using one word at a time, or simple short phrases. Children often misunderstand speech simply because adults talk too fast, not bothering to enunciate the words properly. A flood of quickfire sentences will delay rather than accelerate your child's acquisition of speech, because he will find it hard to distinguish one word from a whole string which sounds to him as if it is all run together. One of my five-year-old pupils had learnt the Lord's prayer at Sunday school but had not been able to pick out the correct words from the chanting of the other children or the teacher who provided the model, and finished with: 'For thine is the kingdom, the power and the laundry, for ever and ever, Amen.' He would not believe me when I tried to point out that it should be, 'the power and the glory', but insisted that this was what they said at *his* Sunday school.

One of the best ways of expanding your child's use of language is to repeat what he has said, in an expanded form. If your two year old says, 'Daddy' and points to the door, you can respond, 'Yes, that's right, Daddy has gone to fetch the car', or, 'Yes, Daddy has gone, but will be back in a minute.' This positive approach works much better than always correcting your child – 'No, say so and so. . . .' Instead, suggest that your child's efforts are right, but by expanding what he has said, show how it could be improved.

At some time between the ages of three-and-a-half and four-and-a-half your child will start to bombard you with an incessant flood of questions about everyone and everything. However many times the same question is asked, and however silly it might seem to you, try to give as full an answer as possible, as the quality of your replies at this stage in his development is believed by experts to be crucial to his intellectual growth. And it is certainly true that a child's eventual linguistic ability depends largely on the standard of his parents' speech, to which he is constantly exposed. So you can't do better than to be as scrupulous as possible when holding conversations around your child – both in your choice of words and in the care with which you say them.

Nursery rhymes

All the old nursery rhymes are invaluable for developing both your child's awareness of words, rhyming and rhythm, and his appreciation of size, length, number, and so on – concepts that often cause confusion for the young dyslexic.

From his first year to third year up your child will enjoy gesture and number rhymes, which will help to lay the foundation for his future numeracy. For example, try reciting the following rhymes, accompanying the words with fingerplay and actions:

Ten little men standing up straight,
Ten little men open the gate,
Ten little men running to play,
Ten little men hiding away.

Or:

One, two, buckle my shoe.
Three, four, open the door.
Five, six, pick up sticks.
Seven, eight, lay them straight.
Nine, ten, a big fat hen.

And, of course, there are other old favourites such as 'Ten Green Bottles', 'This Old Man' and 'Roll Over'.

Toys and other play mediums

Play will not only improve your child's awareness of size, shape and dimension, and speed up his understanding of direction – up, down, right, left, and so forth – but will also help him to become more skilled in other key areas in which dyslexics often lag behind.

Personally, I don't think it is worth buying educational toys for your child before he is two years old. No hard and fast rules can be laid down on this point, but it does seem that a great deal of money is wasted on such toys at an early age when the child would benefit much more from simply exploring his surroundings and playing with everyday items that come to hand. In this way he learns far more about what goes on around him than being swamped by artificially created aids to development.

Give him a wooden spoon with various different types of materials to bash; this is good for hand coordination and will help him learn to distinguish between different sounds. To encourage the use of writing materials give him old newspapers to scribble on. To stimulate his perception of space and direction, provide him with cardboard boxes of different sizes to stack, to get in and out of, and to put things in and take them out again. All these household objects will give hours of useful play without costing a penny.

Most toddlers adore playing with water and you should encourage this whenever possible – bathtime, of course, provides an ideal opportunity. Pouring liquid from one container to another improves hand/eye coordination and with constant practice leads eventually to the understanding that a tall vessel does not necessarily hold more water than a short one – another concept which often foxes dyslexics. Sand is another satisfying and stimulating play medium which helps with the same problems and costs little or nothing. Make sure you buy silver or washed sand rather than the sand builders use, which will stain everything orange. I realize that a great deal of mess can be created with sand and water, but it is well worth while planning how to make them available without ruining the entire home.

Around the time of your child's second birthday, you can usefully expand his opportunities for play with toys bought from a shop. Nowadays there is a bewildering variety of toys on the market and many do not seem worth their exorbitant cost, particularly in terms of their value as educational playthings. If you are worried your child might be dyslexic I would advise you to keep to simple practical toys that will help develop his numeracy, his sense of direction and his skill at playing with two- and three-dimensional shapes. Building bricks are excellent for this (make sure they are solid and large enough to be easily manageable); and so are very simple jigsaws; large, brightly coloured abacuses; sets of large wax crayons; posting boxes with assorted shapes; and towers of different-sized rings on sticks. A tip when buying toys is to check the labelling and packaging to see for what age group they are suitable. This is important because giving your toddler a toy that is meant for an older child might only frustrate him, and could be dangerous if there are small pieces that can be swallowed.

Letters

By the age of four, or as early as his second year, if your child is responsive, you can introduce him to letters. It is easier for him to learn to recognize them than to write them, so, soon after you have begun to familiarize him with their shapes, ask him to pick out a letter from a display. I would recommend beginning with capitals, despite the fact that many school-teachers prefer – wrongly in my view – to start children off on little letters (known as 'lower-case' letters). But if you want to use lower-case letters first, it won't do any harm. First teach him the names of the letters. Again, no expensive equipment is needed. You can show him headlines in newspapers or magazines, or write a few letters – large and clear – on a piece of rough paper.

To make the alphabet more tangible and fascinating, you can buy sets of plastic or wooden letters. These are ideal for playing simple games, like asking your child to bring you one particular letter after another from a jumble of letters on the other side of the room. As he gets to know either the capitals or the lower-case letters, introduce the other form and play games matching the two.

When you are outdoors show him letters on roadsigns and advertisements, and draw his attention to numbers on houses too. Now you can bring in the sounds of letters by discussing their sound at the beginning of each word, as in Car Park or Post Office. Try not to do this if the word has a letter sound at the beginning that does not simply come from one letter – such as Auction Sale. At this stage letter/sound association should be kept simple and regular to avoid confusing your child.

From about the age of three to four you can encourage him to start tracing capital letters. Most children of three should be able to draw a

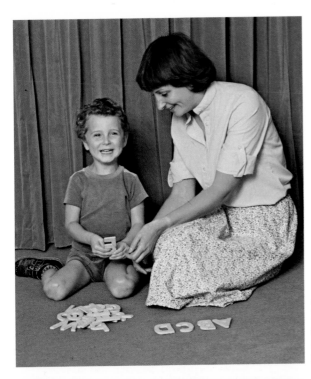

Asking your child to pick out letters from a pile and to say their names aloud is an excellent first step towards learning the alphabet.

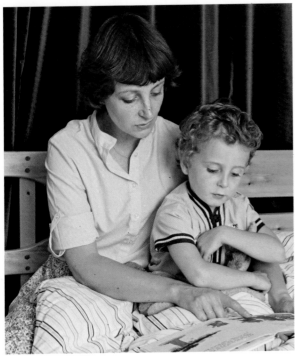

The joy of being read to aloud from a picture book for just five to ten minutes a day at bedtime will stimulate your child's awareness of letters and words, and of graphic shapes and sizes—as well as being an incentive to go to bed!

circle and a straight line, and capitals are composed of a combination of circles or parts of circles, and straight lines. Make sure that he holds the pencil properly (see page 66) and that the letters are correctly formed (see page 68). Once he has mastered tracing, let him move on to copying them freehand.

Books and reading

You can introduce your baby to books even before the end of his first year. Stiff board books with bold colour pictures will stand up to rough handling, and provide entertaining opportunities for introducing him to shapes, directions, counting and matching names to objects – all typical dyslexic problem areas.

Once your child is old enough to understand, try to read aloud to him for five to ten minutes every day. When he is in bed is usually the best time, as he will be more relaxed, and this enjoyable activity provides an incentive for him to go to bed.

Fairy tales with pictures are marvellous first stories. One of the best I know for developing awareness of shapes and sizes is *Goldilocks and the Three Bears.* It contains constant repetition of 'big', 'medium-sized', 'small', 'too high', 'too low', and so forth, which you can make even more meaningful by pointing out details in the pictures and making appropriate gestures.

Illustrated alphabet books are good supplements to the ideas in the previous section for learning letters, and are a first step on the way to proper reading. Particularly effective are the pop-up books where an animal or object will suddenly appear from behind a letter. The more exciting and fun the books, the quicker your child will learn.

If he shows an inclination to read before going to school, by all means encourage this by running your finger under the print as you read and allowing him to follow the line, filling in words as and when he can. If he does not show an interest in books or reading, don't worry or try to force them on him. As I said at the beginning of the chapter, this approach can be counterproductive in the long run, making him bored and resentful. You can be assured that he will get every chance to learn these skills at school, however much difficulty he has with them.

Books on tape These are now very popular with children from the age of four upwards, and many are sold with an accompanying book which you can help your child to follow as the tape is being played. An enormous range of such tapes is now available, from the simplest fairy stories to books for older children, such as *The Hobbit, Watership Down, Tom Sawyer* and scores of other classics that a young dyslexic child might not be able to read for himself. Using books on tape, you will be helping your child to grow up literate, in the sense that he will know about and enjoy literature, even if for a time his literacy skills are not well developed.

How you can help your young schoolchild

If your child is dyslexic, you will almost certainly have noticed some of the symptoms (listed in Chapter 3) by the time he starts formal schooling at around the age of five, and your suspicions should have been aroused. However, a note of caution here: many children starting school make typical dyslexic reading and writing mistakes – letter reversals, and so on – so don't be too worried at this stage. It is generally not until around the age of six and a half that the gap in reading and writing ability between dyslexics and non-dyslexics becomes really noticeable. However, bright children usually begin reading at five, and sometimes earlier. If his teachers agree that your child is continuing to have difficulties while his peers are making good progress, this is the time when efforts should be made to have him expertly assessed (see Chapter 6). Delay, as we have seen, can lead to all sorts of additional problems and it is only once a proper diagnosis has been made that a real start can be made to deal specifically with your child's dyslexia.

What to do if you suspect he is dyslexic

Normally, it is the school who decides that a child needs investigating if he is not progressing well or is presenting a problem in class. In this case, an appointment will be made with the educational psychologist (or school counsellor in Australia) for an assessment and action should be taken with regard to his or her recommendations. Sometimes the action is felt to be unsuitable by the parents, or the school decides to ignore it. Should this happen and you are unhappy about the situation for whatever reason, you should approach the school and make your wishes known. You should also ask for a psychologist's or school counsellor's report if the school has not recognized in the first place that there is a problem which needs investigating.

If neither of these avenues has proved fruitful, it is perfectly possible for you to arrange an independent assessment for your child. In order to do this you can either approach your family doctor, who may refer your child to a reputable psychologist, clinic or hospital known to have special expertise in the field, or you can approach your local dyslexia association (addresses are listed in the Appendix on pages 135–7) for a list of approved names. The former route is probably more reliable, as your family doctor can also arrange appropriate vision and hearing tests and give the psychologist a full picture of your child's general health and family history. On the other hand, dyslexia associations are now very knowledgeable about local facilities for dyslexics, and are specially geared to dealing with these problems.

Of course, if you decide to have your child assessed privately, or you live in a country without a State health service, such as the United States, you can approach a psychologist direct who specializes in learning difficulties such as dyslexia. He should be able to give you a list of suitable teachers, specially trained, who would be able to provide the remedial help that may be needed in addition to anything the school has to offer.

Once dyslexia is diagnosed, it is highly desirable that specialist teaching is arranged to supplement normal school classes. Practice varies widely both nationally and internationally – it is possible that there is a specialist or resource teacher attached to the school, or that one can visit the school regularly; or, there may be a dyslexia clinic or class in your area. If you decide to pay privately for your child's treatment it is important to make sure that the specialist who has been recommended to you has a qualification in dyslexic teaching. Before treatment is started, do ask to see it, and contact your local dyslexia organization if you have any doubts.

Overcoming dyslexia depends on a team effort between the specialist (if one is available), the schoolteacher, the parents and the dyslexic himself. Initially, many of my dyslexic pupils' parents have been unsure of what sort of support they should give their child, and I have often been asked how to help with homework; whether a child would benefit from extra spelling lessons at home; how to prepare a child for the psychological problems he will face; and so on. There certainly are pitfalls in these areas for the inexperienced, but I hope the following guidelines and advice will help you to avoid them and to do the best for your child.

General guidelines for parents
It is not possible to give parents definitive, step-by-step guidelines that are guaranteed to lead to success, as each child will respond differently to whatever is done to help. You should therefore work out by trial and error which of the following approaches and techniques work best in your family.

● Be prepared for your child to be unresponsive to the help you offer. I have found that children are usually more cooperative when their work is given by and accomplished for someone outside the family.

● Whatever your child's attitude, remember that you have a vital role to play in his fight against dyslexia and that your commitment to his progress will probably make all the difference. You have the opportunity to give him the valuable one-to-one attention that he may otherwise lack.

● Try to motivate your child without pressurizing him. Rather than devising extra work at home and continually pointing out his mistakes, spend as much time as you can playing educational games (see pages 52–3), praise even his smallest achievement, and encourage him to build on his strengths as well as to tackle his weaknesses.

● Don't lose your temper if your child is not progressing as fast as you would like, or is slow on the uptake. Overcoming the problems associated with dyslexia can take a long time – and a lot of patient hard work on everyone's part. It is essential that he feels that you are on his side.

● If either you or your child becomes angry or frustrated while working together on reading and writing (as happens in many dyslexics' families), leave practice for a time, until the tensions have eased.

● Keep in touch with his teachers, both his regular schoolteacher and his dyslexia specialist (if he has one). If all of you pool your information, then any problems with your child can be dealt with more effectively. Also, if you decide to give any extra help at home, make sure his teachers know exactly what you are planning to do. Each has his or her own way of working, and should be willing to advise you on what will and what will not fit in with their methods (see Chapter 5).

● Make an effort to meet other parents with dyslexic children. Your local dyslexia organization (see Appendix) may be able to put you in touch with families in your area; or friends and neighbours might well know of others. Swapping information and advice can be very useful, and it will be reassuring to know other people who are managing to cope with similar difficulties to yours.

What practical help can you give?
Once your child goes to school he will get plenty of formal training in the basic techniques of reading and writing. If he is having trouble with them, your first instinct may be to try to give him extra practice at home. By all means continue to read to him as you did before he started school, but don't try to make *him* read every evening unless he wants to. He may be tired and frustrated after a day at school, and any additional pressure might put him off the reading altogether. To encourage him to read of his own accord, find out what he enjoys reading most and have this available at home, even if this means buying him comics. The pictures will at least keep him interested in the written word. There are, though, many other ways in which you can help – remember that by improving his all-round skills, you will also be improving his reading and writing.

With homework Once your child is old enough to be given homework, whether from his schoolteachers or a dyslexia specialist, he will need your assistance with it. Don't simply do it for him – that way he will get no benefit from the work at all. Rather, make yourself available as his 'sounding board'.

Suggest how he might approach the work, try to answer all his questions, and make sure that he double-checks everything. When he has finished, look over what he has done and without actually pointing out his mistakes, ask him if he thinks that he could have expressed this or that better, or that the grammar here or the spelling there could be improved. And don't forget to praise anything he has done well.

With spelling Again, rather than adopting the teacher's role and attempting to make your child learn lists of words, become his companion in a game.

'I Spy' can be played anywhere, any time. Start with the letter name: 'I spy with my little eye, an object beginning with T.' When he has guessed what it is, try again with the letter sound. And finally, when the object is guessed ask your child to try spelling it out.

There are many excellent simple spelling games you can buy, many of which involve letter shapes, letter dice or special cards, but don't be tempted by games as complicated as Scrabble. These are too advanced for a young dyslexic child and if played with the whole family may only make him feel inadequate and inferior.

Depending on your child's age and spelling ability, you might try playing simple crosswords with him, which can be found in puzzle books or children's annuals.

The recently introduced computerized spelling games for children such as Speak and Spell should certainly engage your child's interest if his spelling is sufficiently competent. A voice is programmed to ask the player to type out a simple word. If he gets it wrong, the computer tells him to try again. If he is successful, he will be requested to spell another word. These games are not suitable for children who have difficulty identifying the spoken sounds, because the computerized voice is not sufficiently clear. However, help can be given by an adult and once the word is known, it will be recognized when repeated. In my experience most dyslexics enjoy electronic games and are good at keyboard work, so for around the price of a transistor radio these computer games can be a practical investment.

With sequencing To help with learning the right order of letters in the alphabet, try the following game: Start reciting one letter each alternately, then say three letters each alternately, and finally you say two letters and your child three. This game can also be played with numbers. Games where you join up the dots which are either numbers or letters of the alphabet, resulting in a picture emerging will also help with sequencing. As we have seen, rhymes are good for fixing common sequences in the memory. This gruesome one seems to amuse children and can be used for the days of the week:

Solomon Grundy,
Born on Monday,
Christened on Tuesday,
Married on Wednesday,
Took ill on Thursday,
Worse on Friday,
Died on Saturday,
Buried on Sunday,
This is the end of Solomon Grundy.

When teaching him the order of the seasons and the months, don't just

52

make them seem like boring strings of words to be learned by rote. Get him interested by explaining what happens in them, and relating them to memorable events in his life – winter (if you live in the northern hemisphere), with last Christmas, for instance. The more vivid the mental images you can conjure up, the more likely it is that he will remember their names and hopefully the order.

Good rhymes to improve your child's short-term memory for sequences are 'Old Macdonald Had a Farm', 'This is the House That Jack Built' or 'The Twelve Days of Christmas', all of which gradually build up a long list of items that he will need to remember in the correct order.

With sense of direction Helping your child to sort out which is his left and which his right is obviously your first priority if he has directional confusion. Start off by asking: 'Which is your right eye? Which is your left leg? Which is your right hand?' If he can master this, try asking him which is your own right and left hand when standing opposite him. If he cannot figure this out, try sitting beside him to begin with and asking the same question.

Another popular directional game is 'Simon Says'. Start with a simple instruction like, 'Simon says, "put both hands on top of your head." ' Then gradually make them harder: 'Simon says, "touch your right knee with your left hand," ' and so on. If after endless practice and games, your child still can't remember which hand is which, mark the backs of his hands with a small 'R' and 'L' in ink.

Games such as 'Looby Lou' ('put your right foot in, put your right foot out') and doing mazes will improve your child's sense of direction if you encourage him to say whether he is turning left or right, and the latter will also improve his pencil control. The best way to teach him the points of the compass is to study a map together which features places he is interested in. You can then ask him, for example, in which direction the sea is from your home town.

As I mentioned in the previous chapter, many dyslexic children have difficulty tying their shoe-laces. This too stems from directional confusion as well as lack of dexterity. The best way to deal with this is by daily practice. When showing him the technique it is best to sit facing the same way; if you sit opposite him he may become even more confused. You can buy a toy shoe with laces that comes with very clear instructions and is made specifically for helping dyslexic children with this difficulty. These are available from several educational materials suppliers; your child's school or dyslexia specialist should know where you can buy them.

With telling the time and general organization Not surprisingly, being unable to tell the time from a conventional clock-face and being badly organized at home and school often go together in the dyslexic. A way in which you can attempt to tackle both problems at the same time is to draw

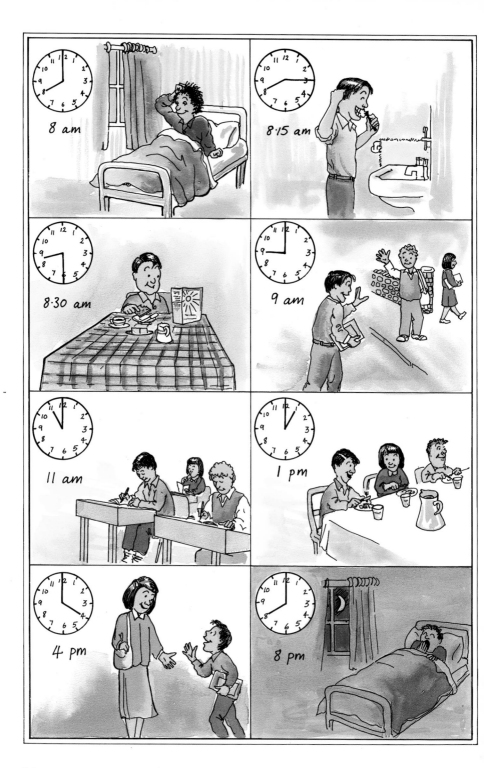

8 am

8·15 am

8·30 am

9 am

11 am

1 pm

4 pm

8 pm

or paint a large wall-chart for your child's bedroom, depicting in step-by-step boxes the different activities of the day in their right order. Each box should be accompanied by a large picture of a clock-face with its hands pointing to the time of day at which the event is supposed to happen. For example, you might draw a child getting out of bed at 8.00 am, a child getting dressed at 8.15 am, having breakfast at 8.30 am, and so on, right through to bedtime.

A wall-chart, though, has its limitations, as each day is never quite the same as the next. So you should always try to be one step ahead when helping your child to organize his routine. Anticipate the problems that are likely to arise and prepare him to cope with them in advance. If, for instance, he is playing in a football match for his school and has to be ready to be picked up by coach, with his things packed, at a certain place and time, you should go over the sequence of events with him several times in the morning until it is fixed in his memory.

General advice to give your child

Relaxed discussion with your young schoolchild about his dyslexia is very important to enable him to cope. For however confident he seems to you, anxieties about his school performance and his relationships with his teachers and fellow pupils are probably never far from the surface. He will need a lot of reassurance that his problem does not mean that he is stupid. You might like to use some of the information you have read in this book to set his mind at rest. The message I try to put across to my dyslexic pupils is: 'Have confidence in yourself. You are just as bright as other children and it's not your fault that reading and spelling are so difficult for you. On the other hand, you may well have to work harder than they do to achieve what you want from life. But this is no bad thing. When you have worked hard for something, you appreciate it so much more than if everything comes easily.'

If you prepare your child for possible taunts about his dyslexia, he will find them easier to deal with. Encourage him to learn to laugh at himself when teased, and to reply with something along the lines of, 'I can't spell, but you can't sing in tune.'

Finally, do explain to him that he should try not to annoy his teachers, as he needs them on his side. But tell him not to be shy to ask for something to be repeated or explained again if he didn't take it in first, second or more times round.

I shall be giving advice for the older dyslexic student in Chapter 8, but it is time now to see what schoolteachers can do to help the dyslexic child.

OPPOSITE: Painting or drawing a daily activity wall-chart for your child's bedroom will help him both to tell the time and to fix in his mind the day's order of events. The aim is that he should eventually become able to organize his day for himself.

5. HOW CAN SCHOOL-TEACHERS HELP?

Although this chapter is aimed chiefly at teachers of five- to twelve-year-old children, the information it contains should also be useful to parents of young dyslexic children, especially if you plan to help your child with his homework. The better informed you are about the methods by which he is likely to be taught at school, the more effectively you can provide home back-up.

I want first to consider the importance of identifying the dyslexic in school, then to explain how schoolteachers can help dyslexics to improve their reading and writing skills in class, and finally to offer some advice on teachers' general approach to dyslexics and on dealing with the everyday problems that are almost certain to arise.

Recognizing dyslexia

Most primary-school teachers will be aware that after the age of around six and a half certain pupils are not progressing as they should with reading and writing, and, accepting that these children might well be dyslexic, arrange for them to be properly tested. The results of not doing so may be disastrous – as Mark's case shows. The following is an excerpt from his teacher's letter, given to me recently by Mark's parents.

> I have conducted a few tests with Mark, and you will be glad to know that he showed no sign whatever of being dyslexic, in fact, he did very well, and made very few mistakes. There is, therefore, no reason at all why he should not radically improve his reading and writing if he makes up his mind to. From talking to him, I have the impression that he rather cherishes the idea of himself as having 'special problems' – his own expression, this – which he seems to think excuse him from making any 'special effort'. I don't believe he has any 'special problem' apart from laziness, and I have told him so. He is an intelligent boy and very plausible and articulate orally, and he has learnt that it requires far less effort to talk his way through things rather than to knuckle down to the disciplines of reading and writing.

Mark was eight years old at the time this letter was written. Four years later he was diagnosed as dyslexic. Now, at the age of sixteen, thanks largely to exceptional hard work and determination, he is about to take his pre-university examinations. Although Mark is extremely intelligent, he is still having great difficulty with spelling, continuing to make many typical dyslexic mistakes (see page 28).

It is of the utmost importance, therefore, that you, as teachers, should not automatically write children off as 'lazy', particularly if they give every sign of being bright in other ways. As I mentioned in Chapter 3, the 'hidden' dyslexic often gives a false impression of being able to read, by learning the reading scheme off by heart.

I know how difficult it can be to give individual attention in the setting of a large class. It is, nevertheless, the teacher's prime responsibility to detect problems early on. This can be done either by testing each child occasionally on unfamiliar reading material, or by conducting a specially developed individual test, such as the Aston Index, or by using a recognized classroom screening procedure, like the Ann Arbor Test. Many education authorities have developed their own screening systems which are usually administered at the age of seven. Once dyslexia is suspected, the teacher should take the appropriate steps to ensure the child is seen by the educational psychologist (or school counsellor in Australia).

However, it is better if dyslexic difficulties in an obviously bright child are detected before this age, as the earlier remedial techniques are begun, the better results they can achieve. We have already seen in Chapter 2 how problems can develop in an undiagnosed dyslexic. His poor written work will cause him to slip further and further behind his peers, resulting either in his having to work with much younger children, or being relegated to remedial classes for all subjects, or, worst of all, being sent to a school for backward children. Needless to say, efforts must be made to avoid these eventualities at all costs.

How schoolteachers can help the dyslexic to improve his reading, spelling and writing

Ideally, a dyslexic child should receive supplementary remedial teaching from a specialist qualified in dyslexic teaching. Unfortunately this is not always possible, and you may be the only professional available to give him guidance with reading and writing. Whatever the situation, his schoolteachers should have a sound knowledge of the principles behind specialist teaching so that they can at least provide suitable back-up for outside tuition. If you can only give five minutes special help a day to dyslexic pupils in class, that might make the difference between their keeping up with their schoolfellows and falling hopelessly behind.

It is not feasible to include my whole dyslexic teaching programme here; that has required a book to itself, namely *Alpha to Omega* (1975). What follows is aimed to show why certain reading systems used in schools may be confusing to the dyslexic, and to give teachers and parents a general idea of the method I favour, by which dyslexics are often successfully taught to read and write. Ideally, the *Alpha to Omega* teaching programme should be used by professionals who have a qualification in dyslexic teaching, but if necessary it can be used by schoolteachers who have not had any specialist dyslexia training, and also by parents, if they read it through carefully beforehand.

Three methods unsuitable for dyslexics

No one knows how a child learns to read, but it seems likely that the skill is picked up by seeing words and hearing them spoken. Eventually the two processes become fused, the written symbols become linked to verbal sounds and print suddenly begins to make sense. For most children this simply 'clicks', for dyslexics it does not.

Initial Teaching Alphabet (ITA)   In an attempt to make bridging the gap between symbol and sound as easy as possible for those learning to read, Sir James Pitman, the British publisher and educationalist (whose relation Sir Isaac Pitman invented the Pitman shorthand method), created the ITA. This is a set of forty-four symbols representing the forty-four sounds of the English language. This system was widely used in Britain during the 1960s and '70s at primary-school level, the intention being that pupils should be switched to the normal alphabet at around the age of seven.

Although brilliantly conceived, the ITA is not as widely used as previously. It has been found that it is not really needed by children who learn to read easily, and eventually confuses dyslexics when they have to make the transition from the ITA and start all over again learning the traditional alphabet – for them a new and different set of symbols.

A dozen lines printed in the Initial Teaching Alphabet explaining about the method which has a different symbol for all forty-four sounds of the English language.

> ꞇhis is printed in an augmented rœman alfabet, ꞇhe purpos ov whiɕ is not, as miet bee suppœsd, tꝏ reform our spelliŋ, but tꝏ imprꝏv ꞇhe lerniŋ ov reediŋ. it is intended ꞇhat when ꞇhe beginner has aɕheevd ꞇhe iniſhal suksess ov flꝏensy in ꞇhis speſhally eesy form, his fuetuer progress ſhꝏd bee konfiend tꝏ reediŋ in ꞇhe present alfabets and spelliŋs ov ꞇhem œnly.
>
> if yꝏ hav red as far as ꞇhis, ꞇhe nue meedium will hav prꝏvd tꝏ yꝏ several points, ꞇhe mœst important ov whiɕ is ꞇhat yꝏ, at eny ræt, hav eesily mæd ꞇhe ɕhænj from ꞇhe ordinary rœman alfabet wiꞇh konvenſhonal spelliŋs tꝏ augmented rœman wiꞇh systematik spelliŋ.

Despite its failure to help dyslexic children read, this bold experiment has taught us one cardinal rule for dyslexic teaching, namely that a child with a learning disability has difficulty in learning, and so nothing should be taught that will later have to be unlearnt.

'Look and Say' Many schools nowadays use a whole-word method of teaching pupils to read, usually known as 'Look and Say'. This is based on the 250 key words that make up most of our speech. By introducing only a few of these words at a time and constantly repeating them – often in association with a picture of the word – it is assumed that children will learn them by sight. Many do, but most dyslexics do not.

When children come across an unknown word, some teachers of the 'Look and Say' method encourage the use of phonics – associating a single letter with a single sound – to help them work it out. The major drawback

The Look and Say method of teaching reading is based upon these 250 key words which make up most of our speech. The whole diagram represents the 20,000 words in an average vocabulary. The frequency of use of the key words is shown by area, and to some extent by the size of the type.

12

a and he
I in is
it of that
the to was

all as at be but are for had have him his not on one said so they we with you 20

about an back been before big by call came can come could did do down first from get go has her here if into just like little look made make me more much must my no new now off only or our over other out right see she some their them then there this two up want well went who were what when where which will your old 68

After Again Always Am Ask Another Any Away Bad Because Best Bird Black Blue Boy Bring Day Dog Don't Eat Every Fast Father Fell Find Five Fly Four Found Gave Girl Give Going Good Got Green Hand Head Help Home House How Jump Keep Know Last Left Let Live Long Man Many May Men Mother Mr. Never Next Once Open Own Play Put Ran Read Red Room Round Run Sat Saw Say School Should Sing Sit Soon Stop Take Tell Than These Thing Think Three Time Too Tree Under Us Very Walk White Why Wish Work Woman Would Yes Year Bus Apple Baby Bag Ball Bed Book Box Car Cat Children Cow Cup Dinner Doll Door Egg End Farm Fish Fun Hat Hill Horse Jam Letter Milk Money Morning Mrs. Name Night Nothing Picture Pig Place Rabbit Road Sea Shop Sister Street Sun Table Tea Today Top Toy Train Water 150

This area represents 19.750 further words. Space does not permit the printing of these words.

with this type of phonic teaching is that it only works when a word's letter/sound associations are totally regular. For example, the word 'bet' can be sounded out with its single letters b/e/t, whereas it is impossible to sound out phonically even such simple, common words as 'her', 'for' and 'car'.

The other flaw in the phonic technique is that letters are usually taught only by their sounds and not their names. This is a big mistake for the following reasons:

1. Many children come to school already knowing the names of the letters and find it confusing to have to call them by something different.
2. Letter names are the only things that are constant. Letter sounds change when used in context in words.
3. Although sounds are essential for reading, names, as I shall be showing, are essential for spelling.

'Language experience' The trend nowadays is to use the child's own language in his reading material. I doubt whether this method will be successful for any pupils, whether dyslexic or not, as all structure for learning goes by the board. And it will certainly not help the socially deprived child to improve his language skills if he is not exposed to anything more advanced than what he is used to hearing at home or among his friends.

A successful teaching system for dyslexics
The structured phonetic/linguistic method is the most effective system used in centres where dyslexics are taught. Unlike the three methods previously described, this one concentrates not just on reading and spelling skills, but also on handwriting and the ability to string words, sentences and ideas together logically. It is preferable to have a thorough knowledge of phonetics (the science of speech sounds) and linguistics (the science of language) in order to teach it. You should not confuse simple phonics with phonetics. Phonics seldom goes beyond the level of single letter to single sound association, whereas phonetics covers the whole range of speech sounds, whether associated with single letters or 'chunks' of letters. Pupils must first be taught the names of the letters in order to learn how 'chunks' of letters sound. To go back to my previous example of the word 'car', which cannot be spelt out by the phonic method, a child must be able to state that the letters 'a' and 'r' are needed to make the sound /ar/. He can then join on the regular sound of the letter 'c' to produce the correct sound: /car/.

From letter names and sounds to words In a structured phonetic/linguistic programme such as *Alpha to Omega* the pupil should be taught logically step by step, beginning with single-letter sounds linked to letter names and letter shapes, and working in stages through simple one-syllable words to complex multisyllabic words. The teaching drills should be based on what specialists term a 'multisensory' technique. In other words, one that utilizes the pupil's senses of sight and hearing, as well as involving writing down and reading back aloud what has been written – an all-round approach that is particularly successful with dyslexics (see page 134).

The method I would recommend for teaching letter/sound associations, as given in the *Alpha to Omega Flashcards,* runs as follows:

1. The teacher presents the letter on a flashcard (these can be drawn if the box of flashcard letters is not available – see below) with the key picture drawn on the reverse side. The pupil should say the letter's name.
2. The teacher says the key word and then the sound of the letter.
3. The pupil repeats key word and sound.
4. The teacher says the sound and then the name.
5. The pupil repeats the sound and gives the name, writing it as he says

An example of the front (below left) and reverse (below right) sides of the flashcards I use to teach letter/sound associations.

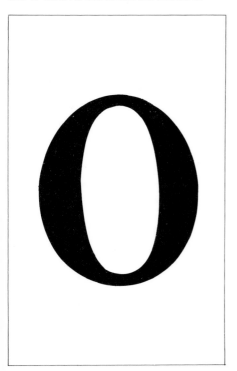
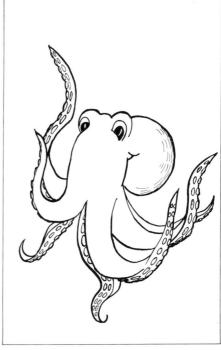

it (translating the sound he has heard into written letters).

6. The pupil reads what he has written, giving the sound (translating the letters written into sounds that are heard).
7. The pupil writes the letter with the eyes closed to get the feel of the letter. (When vision is cut off, other senses, such as touch are sharpened.)

When the child is reasonably familiar with the names, sounds and shapes of the letters, this drill can be modified to:

1. The pupil runs through the flashcards saying their sounds aloud (the reading process).
2. The teacher then dictates each letter sound in random order for the pupil to say the letter's name and then write it down (the spelling process).

This drill should be repeated with each set of new sound patterns shown on the cards. To accelerate reading skill, cards can be given for reading practice that show more advanced patterns than have yet been reached in spelling. This will also help to familiarize the child with the spelling patterns by the time he is expected to spell them.

The association between single-letter name, sound and shape should be taught first, along with the knowledge that some of these letters are vowels, which will be needed in every word. The five basic vowel sounds should then be taught, including the semi-vowel 'y'. 'Y' is more often a vowel than it is a consonant, since it is only a consonant at the beginning of words. Everywhere else in a word, 'y' is a vowel and is used instead of 'i' because no English words end in 'i'. When 'y' is a vowel it has the same sounds as /i/, either long as in 'bȳ' or short as in 'gўpsy'.

The concept of the open and closed syllable needs to be explained to children for them to understand that 'go' does not need to be spelt 'gow'. Since there is not a consonant on the end of the word, the vowel sounds like its name. If the syllable is closed by a consonant, as in 'gŏt' and 'gŏd', the vowel then becomes short. Then all the other nineteen vowel sounds should gradually be revealed in the appropriate spelling pattern, along with the twenty-five consonant sounds.

In order to do this, the pupil has to be introduced to the 'chunking' of consonants and vowels and taught that certain combinations of letters are needed to make certain sounds: 's' and 'h' giving /sh/, for example, 'c' and 'h' giving /ch/ and 't' and 'h' producing either /TH/, the hard or 'voiced' sound as in the word 'the', or /th/, the soft or 'voiceless' sound as in the word 'thin'. Then come the consonant blends, such as 'br', 'pl', 'spr'; and after these the vowel/consonant 'chunks', like 'er', 'or', 'ar', and so on. It is obvious that this is necessary if forty-four sounds are to be represented by only twenty-six letters.

Soon after this the child should be taught that certain letters influence, or modify the vowels that come after them. The letter 'w', for example, changes the sounds of most of the vowels that follow it. Hence 'was' is not spelt 'wos', 'war' is not spelt 'wor', and 'worm' is not spelt 'werm', although the child has just learnt that 'a' is represented by the sounds /ă/ as in 'apple', 'ar' is represented by the /ah/ as in 'car' and /er/ is the sound heard in the word 'her'. The other major modification which has to be taught is the effect that vowels have on the consonants 'c' and 'g', which, when followed by 'e', 'i' or 'y', sound like /s/ or /j/ – as in 'city' and 'gentle', for instance. Of course, there are some extremely common words which do not adhere to this rule, such as 'get', 'girl' and 'gift'; but otherwise it is pretty well followed and helps with reading as well as spelling.

Gradually you should cover the complete range of spelling patterns, culminating in the final syllables 'tion', 'sion', 'cian', 'tial', 'cious', 'cient', 'tient', 'cial' and so on. The English language contains many such oddities and irregularities that have to be explained to the dyslexic. You can perhaps now better appreciate why such a detailed knowledge of phonetics is desirable if this system is to be taught successfully.

From words to sentences   Dyslexics find it hard to form sentences using the words they have learnt. So in addition to having a thorough knowledge of phonetics and English spelling patterns, it would be advisable for the teacher to understand about the structure of language and how it develops. Dyslexic pupils should be introduced by dictation to sentence formation in its simplest form as described by the famous American linguist Noam Chomsky, who believes that all language is stored in the brain in simple, active, affirmative, declarative (SAAD) sentences. Examples of SAAD sentences are:

The man ran to the red van.
A black cat jumped onto the table.

Note, however, that you must match the phonetic content of sentences to your pupils' level. The first sentence above could be introduced at an early stage because it contains phonically regular words, whereas the second sentence features many spelling and sound patterns that may not have been taught. For instance:

● The consonant blend /bl/ at beginning of the word 'black'.
● The 'ck' ending which is only used in one-syllable words without another consonant before the final /k/ sound (as in 'bank').
● The spelling of the regular past tense 'ed', which never sounds like /ed/.
● The final syllable 'ble' which has a sound similar to /bull/, in the word 'table'.

The method I use for dictating sentences is again based on the multisensory technique – involving the pupil in listening, speaking, writing, seeing and reading.

1. Dictate the whole sentence as you would normally say it.
2. Ask the pupil to repeat it aloud.
3. Dictate it again, isolating each word and speaking very clearly so that he does not hear the words run together in strings, but separated, as they will be written down (making the translation from spoken to written language).
4. The pupil writes the sentence, saying it clearly as he writes it (he is now making the translation from spoken to written language for himself).
5. Ask pupil to read aloud exactly what he has written.
6. Suggest final corrections if the pupil fails to discover them for himself. Never tell him what he should have written, rather lead him by appropriate clues to find out for himself, and encourage him to make double-checking of all his work second nature.

This method also increases the child's memory for sentences, as you start with short sentences and progress to increasingly long ones. In their basic form, all ideas exist in the mind as SAAD sentences, and are changed into a more appropriate and complicated structure to convey the required meaning. So once the dyslexic pupil has mastered simple SAAD sentences, the next step is to practice turning them into progressively more sophisticated expressions. The phonetic content of these sentences can be made more difficult as the pupil progresses.

1. **The SAAD sentence:** 'A rat is a pet.'
2. **The question** – but only at the simple reversal of verb level: 'Is a rat a pet?' More difficult types of question structures should only be introduced much later on – the tag question, for example. This can be either a negative tag to a positive statement: 'It is a nice day, isn't it?', or a positive tag to a negative statement: 'It isn't a nice day, is it?'
3. **The negative,** only at the simple level of dropping in the word 'not'. 'A rat is not a pet', for example. Note that the negative can be difficult for dyslexics both to understand and produce. A sentence like: 'Twenty-one is not an even number', may well cause confusion.
4. **The compound sentence** – one consisting of more than one principal clause, as in: 'The cat can sit on my lap, but that dog cannot.' ('Sit on my lap' is understood in the second clause.)
5. **The negative question,** with or without tags. For instance: 'It isn't fun to run in the wet, is it?'

6. **The complex sentence**, one consisting of a principal clause and one or more subordinate clauses – 'The man, who wore a leather coat, hit the dog.'
7. **Cause and effect** 'I would have liked to have gone to the concert, but it would have made me late for my train.'
8. **The passive** 'The dog was beaten by the man in the leather coat.'
9. **The negative passive** 'The dog was not beaten by the man in the leather coat, but by a cruel boy.'

Breaking up word strings   You will need to make it clear to the dyslexic how words change when they are used in everyday speech. We do not write out sentences as we speak because in speech the words are run together into strings. When writing down what we say and hear, we have to be able to break up this flow of sound into isolated words. Dyslexics, as I have mentioned previously, often do not understand this and will write such things as, 'I came to school smorning', even at the age of fourteen. This is how they hear the sentence, so you need to explain first how the words are split – 'this morning'; and then how the word is used in other contexts – 'that morning', 'the other morning'. The dyslexic can only learn to break up the verbal strings of speech correctly by writing practice. Handwriting, of course, is a major stumbling block for many dyslexics, and you should adopt the same clear, logical approach to the teaching of this skill also.

Handwriting and letter forms

I do not want to try to lay down any hard-and-fast rules about teaching handwriting to dyslexics, as this is largely dictated by the policy of the school, your own preference and the child's degree of pencil control. However, I hope the following advice will prove successful when you are teaching a child who has seemingly insoluble difficulties in this subject. Many of the common problems that arise, such as the confusion between 'b' and 'd' can be sorted out if the right approach is taken.

Basic handwriting technique
The best first writing implement for the dyslexic is a medium-soft (HB or No 2) pencil. Corrections can be made with an eraser and pencil is not as messy as ink to start with. As he becomes more competent, he can begin to use a pen. A fountain pen is better than a ballpoint for promoting good letter formation as it has to be held correctly for the nib to work at all. Left-handed nibs can be obtained for left-handers. The correct grip should be encouraged from the start (see overleaf), as bad habits are very difficult to rectify later on – rather like a poor golf swing.
   The pencil should be held lightly to avoid becoming tense and tired, and

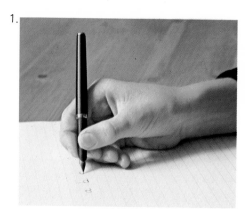

1.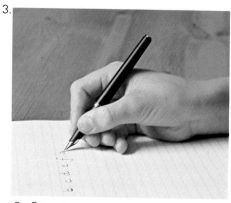

1. Angle of pen too high.

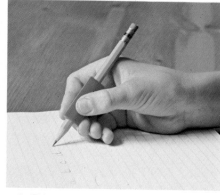

2. Angle of pen too low.

3.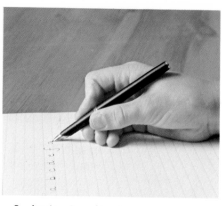

3. Correct pen angle.

4. Triangular plastic grips help to position fingers correctly.

6. Typically dyslexic left-handed 'hook' grip.

5. Typically dyslexic 'fist' grip.

5.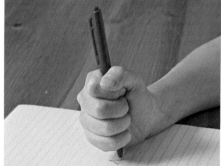

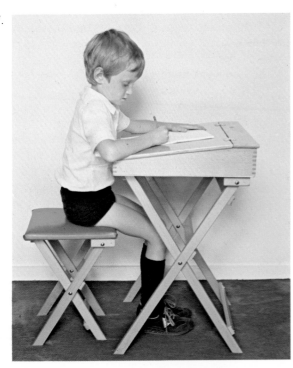

7. The correct seating position for handwriting: elbows resting at right angles on the desk, feet flat on the floor and back straight.

8. The paper should be slanted to the right for the left-hander, and be positioned further to one side than for right-handers so their writing hand does not have to cross the mid-line extending from the nose and obscure what they are writing.

9. For the right-hander, the paper should be slanted to the left, and be positioned closer to the mid-line than for the left-hander.

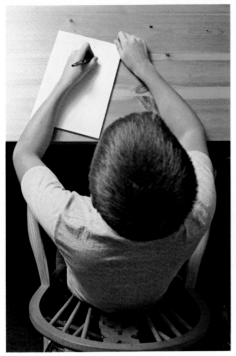

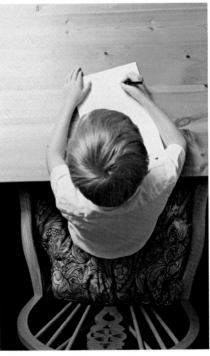

plastic pencil grips will help to achieve the best positioning of the fingers on the pencil (see page 66). With the older pupil it may not be possible to change the grip, only to improve his handwriting.

The child should be comfortably seated, with the desk and chair at the right height so that his elbows rest at right-angles on the writing surface, his back is straight, and his feet flat on the floor (see previous page).

The paper should be slanted to the right for the left-handed writer and to the left for the right-hander. And make sure the paper is further to the left for the left-handers so that their writing hand does not have to cross the mid-line and obscure the pencil point from view as it writes (see previous page). The other hand should rest on the paper to hold it in place – the head does not need supporting, it can support itself! Many dyslexics have problems keeping their letters in a straight line, so it is preferable to use ruled paper for writing practice.

Forming the letters

As I pointed out in the previous chapter, most children can draw circles and straight lines by the age of three and a half. Even if they develop these skills late, as some dyslexics do, there are few who cannot draw lines and circles by the time they start school.

Capital letters are composed of straight lines and circles, or parts of circles, although the lines and curves have to be properly orientated (see below); I see no harm, therefore, in the teacher starting a child off on capitals, as they are easier and more natural for him to form than little or lower-case letters. To begin with they can be written as large as he likes. Some infant teachers object to teaching capitals first, because of the risk that children might then use them wrongly. This will not happen, of course, if they are taught when and where to use them.

The first step is to ask him to trace the letters, then to copy them freehand, and finally to draw them from memory. Once the capitals have been mastered, you can begin to teach the lower-case letters. Many schools teach so-called 'ball and stick' or 'golf club' letters, which are also based on simple circles or parts of circles and straight lines (see opposite, above). I do not recommend teaching this type of manuscript handwriting to

A first capital alphabet suitable for copying.

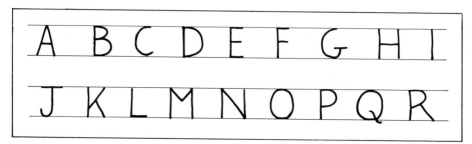

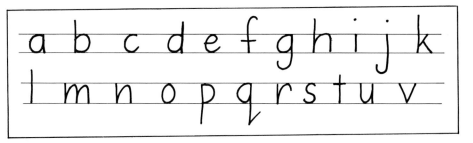

A 'ball and stick' lower-case alphabet—not recommended for dyslexics.

dyslexics because many of the letters are too easily confused – particularly 'b' and 'd' – and difficulties occur when they make the changeover to cursive, or joined-up writing.

Even some of the 'ball and stick' letters cannot be drawn without a curve on either the ascender, as in 'f', or on the descender, as in 'g' and 'j', so it seems a pity not to have ligatures, or curved linking strokes, on all the letters as in the modified cursive style immediately below. Then the child only has to extend these linking strokes to produce joined-up writing, rather than having to relearn all his letter shapes. In my experience, this is the most successful style for dyslexics.

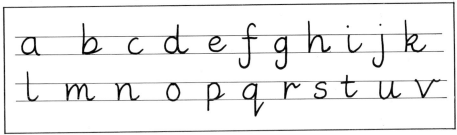

A modified cursive alphabet—in my opinion the best for dyslexics.

Some specialists, though, believe that fully cursive writing should be taught from the start (see below). These are the letter forms the child will eventually use, the style is quicker when it is mastered, will lead to better handwriting in later years, and creates a feeling of flow from the beginning

A fully cursive alphabet, with word examples.

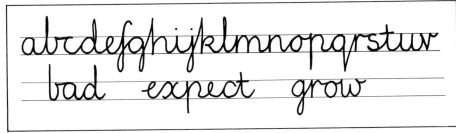

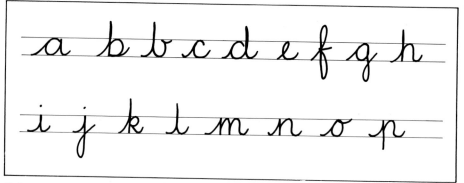

Fully cursive letters in isolation, starting on the base line.

of a word to the end and from left to right along the line. It also sometimes helps with confusions on 'b' and 'd', and 'p' and 'q'.

However, I do not advocate teaching fully cursive letters in isolation if every letter is then started on the base line (see above). This is because when letters are used in context in a word, not all of them will start from the base line. Note that in the example below (top), neither does the 'i' in 'wind' start from the base line, nor the 'o' and the second 'b' in 'bob', nor the 'v' nor the 'e' in the word 'cover'. If the child tries to write these words with all letters commencing from the base line, as he has been taught to do, a most curious effect will be produced – as you can see in the examples below (bottom). You will note that the 'w' has been extended so that it looks like an upside down 'm', two extra strokes have had to be inserted before and after the 'b's in 'bob', which give the appearance of 'i's, the 'o' in 'cover' has now become an 'a' and, again, it looks as though there is an 'i' before the 'e'. I have actually seen dyslexic children writing words like this.

The other objection to teaching all letters starting from the base line is

TOP: Fully cursive letters do not always start from the base line. BOTTOM: The same words with every letter starting from the base line.

wind   bob   cover

wind   bob   cover

70

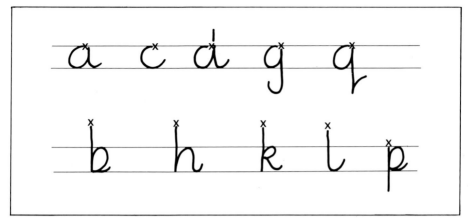

Letters should be taught in groups with similar starting points, here marked with an 'x'.

that the dyslexic loses the important clues about where letters do in fact start, which would help him to appreciate the differences between similar-shaped letters. If letters are taught in groups as shown above so that the child knows that 'd' will start in the same place as 'a', 'c', 'g', 'q', and so on, while 'b' will start at the top like an 'h', it often helps to resolve the intractable problem of 'b' and 'd' confusion. I have yet to meet a child who reverses 'h', so this is a good letter to start with when teaching 'b'. This lack of reversal on 'h' is possibly due to the fact there is not a similar letter that faces the other way, although 'h' is often inverted into a mirror-written 'y', particularly when a 'ball and stick' 'h' has been taught.

Of course, it can be argued that 'b' and 'd' will often start from the base line, according to the context of the letters preceding them. Nevertheless, it is important for the child to realize and aim for the correct starting point for each letter in order to avoid reversing them, even though he is using cursive. I have known several dyslexic children who produced the most beautiful cursive writing and yet still consistently reversed 'b' and 'd' because they had not been taught the vital starting point for each letter.

Which typeface is easiest to read?
Arguments similar to those about handwriting also apply when considering which is the easiest printed typeface for dyslexics to read. Many teachers choose early reading books set in manuscript, or 'ball and stick' type because it looks most like the writing style the child is using. In my view, this is a mistake as the letters in manuscript type can be easily confused, being sans serif – that is, without little tops or bottoms to letters. Times New Roman, a typeface with serifs, has been shown to be the most easily read print. It would be impossible, of course, to ensure that every early reading book for your dyslexic pupils is set in this particular typeface, but I feel strongly that teachers should try to provide books set in a serif face – as this one is – whenever possible.

Helping dyslexics in class

There are many important points that you will need to bear in mind when handling a dyslexic pupil, other than the sheer mechanics of the educational method you are using.

Sit him at the front of the class
If possible, have the child sit at the front of the class rather than leaving him day-dreaming and neglected at the back. It will then be possible to keep an eye on him to ensure that he has understood what is being taught, feels he is receiving attention, and can be given different work from the rest of the class if necessary, without letting everyone know. You can also check that anything written on the board has been correctly copied and give help if it has not.

Speak clearly
Dyslexic children are often very sensitive to loud aggressive voices and respond poorly to teachers who shout at the class – whether because they are angry or because they think that the louder they talk, the better the pupils will understand. Unless you speak very slowly, clearly and calmly, carefully enunciating every word, dyslexics are unlikely to pick up anything at all. Why not take a leaf from presenters of language-learning programmes on radio and television, who keep their sentences short, speak each one in a very clear voice, constantly repeating in different contexts the words to be learnt.

Write clearly
Teachers' handwriting is not always all that easy to read, and particular attention should be paid to writing clearly on the board, and making legible corrections in the child's book. Always write large enough on the board for the whole class to be able to read and do not then stand in front of the board so that nobody can see.

Make allowances
If the dyslexic's written school work is judged on the same criteria as his peers', he will always be seen to be lagging behind. It can take a dyslexic child hours of hard work to produce just a few lines of passable writing, and there can be nothing so demoralizing for a keen young pupil as to feel that all his effort counts for so little.

The teacher's role should be to praise his effort even though the results seem poor in comparison to non-dyslexics' work, and to encourage him to improve on his own performance in subjects requiring literacy skills, rather than to be always competing with children who in his eyes may seem to have an unfair advantage. The answer, as we have seen, does not lie in placing the dyslexic pupil in a remedial class for all school subjects or in removing him to a special school – except in extremely severe cases. Instead, you should make certain allowances for him in class, treading a tightrope between not giving him enough special attention on the one hand, and overdoing it on the other, to the point where he is made to feel like an outsider among his own classmates. Achieving the right balance requires fine judgement based on an awareness of what measures are likely to work for which pupils. In my experience, the following suggestions have often been helpful in successfully integrating a young dyslexic into the school routine.

● Give the dyslexic more time than the other children to produce written work in class and expect less in terms of quantity. Give him easier work than the rest of the class, and when assessing the quality of his work, mark for content rather than presentation. The same rules of thumb apply when writing end-of-term reports and assessments.

● If you feel sufficiently at home with phonetics and linguistics to give the dyslexic tuition along the lines that I described earlier in this chapter, then you should set this sort of work while the rest of the class is engaged in orthodox reading, writing and spelling exercises.

● When marking the dyslexic's written work do not pepper the paper with red correction marks. These will only confuse him and sap his self-confidence, and are extremely unlikely to lead to any improvement. It is more helpful to draw his attention to perhaps three or four mistakes, preferably in phonetically similar words, such as 'park', 'start' and 'bark', and ask him to learn these for next time. A little concrete progress is better than none at all. Note that it will be of little value to point out groups of thematically associated words, like 'butcher', 'postman' and 'dentist', that bear no relation to each other phonetically.

● Involve the dyslexic verbally as much as possible in the classroom to compensate for his lack of literacy skills. More than likely, he will know the answers to questions and take pride in showing off his knowledge to the rest of the class – a great confidence booster. However, there is nothing so terrifying for the dyslexic as to be asked to read aloud in class, so spare him this ordeal and leave oral reading practice either for the extra time you can spare him on his own, or for his specialist teacher to organize.

● Try not to overload the dyslexic with homework. He will probably take much longer over it than his fellows, and unless allowances are made he will have no time for other things. To help him cut down on homework time, ask him to produce work on tape, if he has access to a tape recorder at home. This will give him a chance to display his creativity in an enjoyable medium that should hold no fears.

● As we have seen, the dyslexic child is likely to have problems organizing himself and his belongings, so try not to get as irritated with him as with other pupils if he turns up with his paintbox for a history lesson, or fails to appear at all because he has gone to the wrong classroom or has been unable to tell the correct time. Be lenient over sloppy appearance too. If

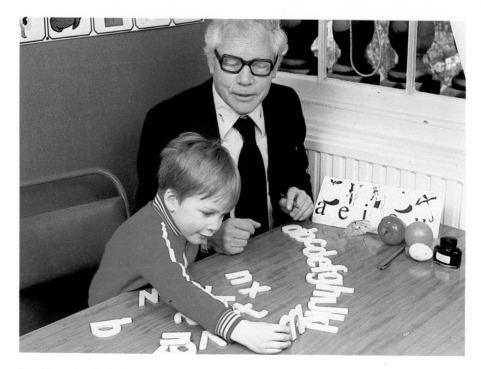

Teaching the dyslexic child demands all a schoolteacher's professional skill. But it is seldom that months of hard, individually tailored work do not bring results.

his shoe-laces are always undone and his tie stuck in a granny knot at half-mast, this is probably due to a genuine difficulty rather than laziness. Patiently keep pointing out what's wrong, and showing him how to put it right, and the penny will drop eventually.

It cannot be denied that the dyslexic pupil places enormous demands on his schoolteachers. To cope effectively requires intelligence, humour, flexibility, sensitivity, empathy, endless patience and preferably a very sound knowledge of what is being taught and why. However, one of the most rewarding aspects of teaching dyslexics is that the majority have the intelligence, enthusiasm and ability to do well if handled in the right way, and there can be nothing more professionally satisfying than to see months or years of hard work come to fruition, as it often does when dyslexia is recognized early enough and the appropriate kind of teaching is given. The key to successful dyslexic teaching is neatly summed up in this ancient Chinese proverb:

We hear, we forget.
We see, we remember.
We do, we understand.

74

6. PROFESSIONAL DIAGNOSIS: TESTS YOUR CHILD MIGHT BE GIVEN

As I have stressed many times throughout the book, professional diagnosis is the first step on the road to appropriate teaching and hopefully to recovery for the dyslexic. Normally this is carried out by a psychologist (or school counsellor in Australia) or medical doctor who specializes in learning disorders such as dyslexia, and depending on your circumstances, your child might be referred for diagnosis by his school, a speech therapist or his family doctor, or you might approach a specialist direct who has been recommended by your doctor, a teacher, a parent of a dyslexic, or your local dyslexia association (see Appendix for addresses).

He will carry out a range of different tests which should enable him to tell whether your child is dyslexic or if there are some other factors that may be hindering his progress at school, such as a low IQ, or physical or emotional illness. The results should also confirm which typically dyslexic problems your child suffers from, to what extent they affect him, and could give an idea of how long it might take before your child's reading and writing is brought up to an acceptable level by remedial teaching.

The psychologist who examines your child may use some or all of the tests mentioned in this chapter, or others that have not been included. Don't be alarmed if the techniques are not exactly the same as I have described here. These are the ones I generally use, but each psychologist has his own preferred way of working and will know which procedures are best for your child. Do ask him to explain anything you don't understand.

All such tests should only be performed by professionals. It is very important that you should not try to use any of the procedures to reach a do-it-yourself diagnosis – without the necessary background knowledge it is easy to misinterpret the results and arrive at completely the wrong conclusion. Bear in mind also that the following tests are for children between the ages of six-and-a-half and sixteen – different ones are needed for younger or older people, but the vast majority of those seen for assessment fall within this age group.

I usually carry out all the tests in one morning or afternoon. Some psychologists, though, prefer to see a child on several occasions for a longer assessment. And there are some tests the psychologist will want performed later by other specialists. However long the process takes, fear of the unknown can make the visit a frightening prospect for a youngster. Understanding what the tests are and what they are designed to show will enable you to explain to your child in advance what he might be asked to do, and reassure him that there is nothing to worry about. If possible, arrange with the psychologist that you should accompany your child, this way he will be more at ease, not only making it less of an ordeal, but also helping him to perform up to his normal standard. If he is tense and upset during the tests, the results obviously won't reflect his true ability.

Tests that are usually given at an assessment

General intelligence test

The most common IQ test for assessing possible dyslexics is known as the Wechsler Intelligence Scale for Children (WISC). This was originally developed in the United States, but is now used around the world. It is ideally suited to children with reading and spelling difficulties because it involves no reading and writing at all. For this reason it is far better than group intelligence tests, often given in the classroom, which depend largely on a child's literary ability.

Like most intelligence tests, this one is split into two halves. One aims to assess your child's intellect by what he can say about things and the other to test what he can do in visual and manual tasks that require no speaking. The test is divided in this way because verbal skill is generally governed by the left half of the brain, and visual and manual performance by the right half. Most people score equally well or equally badly in both sets of tests, so if there is a big difference between your child's verbal and non-verbal, or 'performance', ability, this will show that one half of his brain is working very much better than the other (see Chapter 9). This kind of imbalance will throw the learning process out of true and can result in learning difficulties such as dyslexia.

Verbal test 1: Information   This is aimed to assess your child's range of general information and knowledge of the world around him, as well as his memory for facts which he may have learnt at school. Questions might range from, 'What does a horse eat?', to, 'What is the highest mountain in the world?'

Verbal test 2: Comprehension   This tests his practical judgement, common sense and awareness of why things are done as they are. Questions might range from, 'What would you do if you had a nosebleed?', to, 'Why do we have to pay taxes?'

Verbal test 3: Arithmetic   Here he will be given mental arithmetic problems to test his arithmetic ability, concentration and memory. All the questions can be worked out by common sense, without any specialized knowledge of mathematics.

Verbal test 4: Similarities To check his abstract reasoning, he will be asked in what way pairs of things are alike. To begin with, the similarities should be obvious, as in questions like, 'In what way are a potato and a carrot alike?' The questions then get progressively harder, up to the level of say, 'How are 398 and 677 alike?'

Verbal test 5: Vocabulary This test normally gives the best pointer to your child's intelligence. He will be asked to define a number of words, the questions ranging in difficulty from, for example, 'What is a cow?', to, 'Can you tell me what "ubiquitous" means?'

Verbal test 6: Digit span The examiner will say out loud a random sequence of numbers, and ask your child to repeat them both forwards and backwards. Although his score on this test will not be used to calculate his IQ, it provides useful information about his attention and memory for numbers – lack of which is a possible pointer to dyslexia.

If on the day of the assessment your child won't respond verbally to these tests because he is too shy, or upset, or is just having an off day, other tests can be substituted for the verbal half of the WISC. The psychologist can get a very good idea of your child's vocabulary level merely by asking him to single out one picture from a group, which most nearly matches words spoken aloud by the examiner.

Performance test 1: Picture completion All the performance tests are timed. The first is designed to find out how good your child is at distinguishing the essential details of a picture. He will be asked to say what is missing from a series of drawings – a face without a nose, or a car without a wheel, for example.

Performance test 2: Picture arrangement This will test his skill at sizing up situations and his understanding of cause and effect. The examiner will ask him to arrange a mixed-up sequence of pictures in the right order to make a sensible story – for instance, a drawing of a big splash in a swimming pool, a man poised on a diving board and a man with wet hair towelling himself down.

Performance test 3: Block design To test his spatial ability and eye/hand coordination he will be asked to make patterns with blocks to match patterns shown in a booklet.

Performance test 4: Object assembly This is for assessing similar skills to the previous test. He will be asked to assemble parts of an object – a house, perhaps – into a whole. He is told what the object is supposed to be in the first two items but has to guess for himself in the last two.

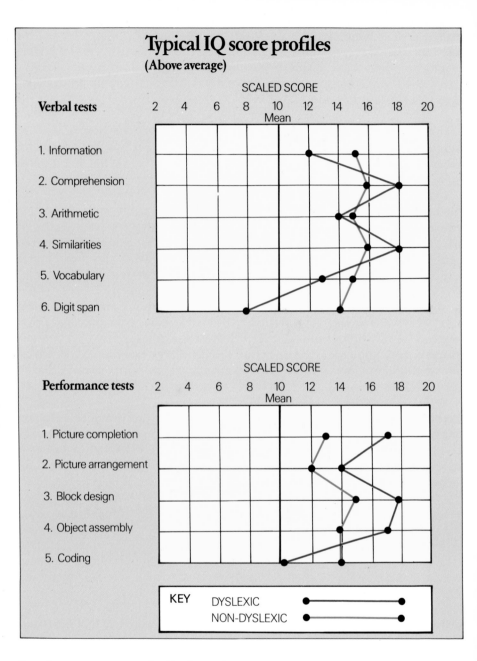

Typical IQ score profiles
(Above average)

Verbal tests

SCALED SCORE

| | 2 | 4 | 6 | 8 | 10 Mean | 12 | 14 | 16 | 18 | 20 |

1. Information
2. Comprehension
3. Arithmetic
4. Similarities
5. Vocabulary
6. Digit span

Performance tests

SCALED SCORE

| | 2 | 4 | 6 | 8 | 10 Mean | 12 | 14 | 16 | 18 | 20 |

1. Picture completion
2. Picture arrangement
3. Block design
4. Object assembly
5. Coding

KEY   DYSLEXIC

NON-DYSLEXIC

Based on my own research, this shows the average scores of dyslexics and non-dyslexics on the tests which make up the Wechsler Intelligence Scale for Children or WISC (see previous two pages). Each group has its own typical profile, which is shown by the shapes of the interconnecting lines. Very significant clues for the diagnosis of dyslexia are the low scores on the Digit Span and Coding tests. These indicate a lack of short-term memory for abstract symbols, shapes and numbers.

Performance test 5: Coding This is a speed test of your child's fine muscular coordination, and his ability to learn a new task and to translate numbers into symbols. For example, a code is given in which shapes or numbers are matched to signs, and your child will be asked to fill in the appropriate sign when shown only the shape or the number.

How IQ is calculated Taking into account your child's age, a scaled score will be calculated for each of the tests, ranging from 0–20 or sometimes 0–19, the average for each test being 10. The scaled scores, apart from Digit Span, are then added up and converted using statistical formulae into a verbal IQ and a performance IQ. The full-scale IQ is a statistical conversion of the sum total of all the verbal and performance scaled scores, apart again from Digit Span. Most people have full-scale IQs of between 90 and 109 (see diagram below). It is currently becoming unpopular in some quarters to talk about intelligence levels or quotients, but there is really no other objective way of assessing what could be expected of a child, and is certainly useful when deciding whether a child should be placed in a school for the educationally subnormal or not.

This shows the percentages of children who fall into each IQ range. Half are in the Average range—with an IQ of between 90 and 109.

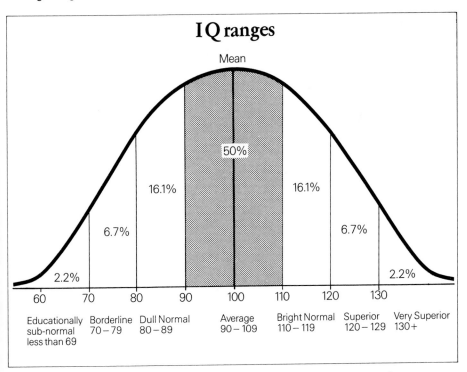

A reading test

The psychologist will give your child one from a number of different reading tests that are available. The one I use is called the Neale Analysis of Reading Ability. I first ask the child to read aloud from a set text and then ask him to give me verbal answers to several comprehension questions. This test takes from ten minutes to half an hour, depending on how far the child can progress. The Neale Analysis is probably the most comprehensive reading test, as it gives not only an accuracy reading age for your child, but also a comprehension reading age and a speed reading age.

There are numerous other tests which are very good. In some, your child will be asked to read aloud from a list of increasingly difficult isolated words, in others he will need to write down his answers to comprehension questions or fill in words that are missing from the text.

When assessing the work, the psychologist will not just be interested in the level of your child's reading ability, but also in the type of mistakes he is making. If he constantly confuses words which look similar, leaves the endings off words, loses his place, reads the same phrase or line twice, mixes up the order of syllables in a word, swops round letters in a word ('clamness' for 'calmness', for instance), or reads words backwards ('saw' as 'was', and 'on' as 'no'), or misreads letters such as 'b' for 'd', or 'n' for 'u', these will be strong pointers to dyslexia.

A spelling test

Again, there is a wide variety of tests from which the psychologist can choose. Most of them are designed to discover your child's spelling age and are given by dictation. I use the Midland Spelling Test because it is less familiar to schoolteachers, which means that the words in the test will probably not have been practised before. I dictate groups of five words, one at a time, each group more difficult than the last. The child's reading age can be calculated from the level at which he spells all the words correctly, before failing on three consecutive words in the level above. This all takes from between five to ten minutes.

Other spelling tests require a child to make between eight and ten errors before testing ceases. Most spelling tests present words of increasing difficulty, like the Midland Test, although there are some which aim not to give a spelling age but to find out the particular areas where your child has problems.

Sequencing tests

Dyslexic children, as I mentioned in Chapter 3, often have trouble placing things in the right order, so the examiner will carry out several short tests to see if your child has noticeable difficulties of this sort. He might ask him to repeat numbers forwards and backwards, to memorize shapes and reproduce them in a certain order, or to recite the alphabet, the months of the year or multiplication tables.

Tests for directional confusion

Again, the majority of dyslexics often confuse right with left, up with down and so forth. The examiner may ask your child to touch his own right leg or ear, to touch his right eye with his left hand, to walk across the room and make a right turn or a left turn, and to point out the right and left sides of the person sitting opposite him. If your child has directional confusion, these tests will almost certainly bring it to light.

Tests to discover his preferred hand and eye

These are important because many typically dyslexic problems are the result of having the preferred, or dominant hand on the opposite side to the preferred eye. People who are right-handed have a natural tendency to write from left to right, while those who are left-handed, to write from right to left. Those who are right-eyed have a natural tendency to scan the page from left to right and those who are left-eyed, to scan from right to left. If you are what is termed a 'crossed lateral', that is, right-handed and left-eyed or vice versa, obviously there will be a degree of confusion between the direction in which your hand wants to write and that in which your eye wants to read. Many people's brains learn to cope successfully with this conflicting information, and so not everyone who is a crossed lateral is dyslexic. However, around 45 per cent of dyslexics are crossed lateral.

Merely knowing that your child writes with his right hand does not necessarily mean that he is right-handed. If he is ambidextrous, he will probably have a preferred hand, say his right, for jobs requiring one hand, like writing, and perform actions that need two hands left-handed – such as eating or playing golf. So at the assessment he will be asked to carry out a series of simple tasks, both single-handed – writing or cutting with scissors, for example – and double-handed, like dealing cards or unscrewing a jar. If he performs all of them either right-handed or left-handed and that hand is also the stronger he will have a clearly preferred hand and cannot therefore be ambidextrous.

In simple terms, your child's preferred, or dominant eye is the one that 'controls' his seeing, leading the other eye to whatever it is he wants to look at; and it is easy for the examiner to find out which your child's preferred eye is. He may either ask him to take a card with a hole in the middle in both hands, to bring it close to his face and look through the hole – the eye he uses will be his preferred eye. Or he may ask him to look through a tube held at arm's length, both eyes open, at an object on the floor. The examiner will then cover each eye in turn. When the preferred eye is covered, the object will seem to vanish; when sight to the other eye is blocked off, the object will remain visible in the tube. Your child may also be asked to sight with a rifle or to look through a telescope. The preferred eye is not necessarily the 'better' eye for sharpness of vision.

Case history

No assessment would be complete without a full case history being taken. This will help the psychologist either to spot possible conditions other than dyslexia that might account for your child's reading and writing difficulties, or to get a better idea of what might have caused his dyslexia. He will ask you for details about the following:

1. Your child's birth and the preceding pregnancy.
2. The ages when your child first performed certain skills, such as walking, talking, holding a pencil properly, and so on.
3. Whether any other members of your family have had dyslexic problems, or whether there is a history of left-handedness, ambidexterity, speech defects or of any other illness in the family.
4. Whether you have noticed anything unusual or worrying in your child's behaviour.
5. Your circumstances at home.
6. Your child's school performance.

It is a good idea to jot down notes beforehand on these points, so you can give the psychologist as full an account as possible. This is important, as even details you might not think are relevant, may give him important clues.

The tests described so far form the basic core of an assessment for dyslexia. There are others, though, which may be given, depending on the way in which the examiner works, and your child's performance so far.

Tests that are sometimes given at an assessment

Passage of free writing

If your child is dyslexic, a five-minute piece of composition, written without any help from the examiner and without any guidance on what he should write about (unless your child is totally unable to think of a theme for himself), will reveal many mistakes which will not have shown up on the standard spelling tests mentioned earlier (see page 80). Although in the previous spelling test he may already have confused 'b', 'd' and 'p', put letters in the wrong order in words, spelled words exactly as they sound or have spelled words bizarrely, the free-writing test will give the examiner a much broader view of his dyslexic difficulties. It will show up deficiencies in his punctuation, sentence structure and grammar, as well as in his handwriting and his ability to keep words in a straight line on unlined paper. This is an optional test, but one that I find very useful and nearly always ask the child to perform.

Tests for perception of sight and sound

These are designed to see how well your child's brain interprets the sights and sounds he sees and hears. Although his sight and hearing may be perfectly normal, he may have difficulty making sense of what he sees and hears. I like to carry out these tests at every assessment – they take around ten minutes to perform – but many psychologists prefer not to unless the child's behaviour or performance suggests that they are necessary.

Your child's visual perception can be tested in various ways, but most probably by a shape-copying test known as the Bender-Gestalt Test. He will be asked to copy nine simple designs composed of lines or dots, which are shown to him one at a time on cards (see page 98).

His perception of word sounds will be checked in the following way. To avoid lip-reading, the examiner will stand behind your child's back and read aloud one at a time a specially prepared list of around twenty to forty pairs of words, some different but sounding alike – like 'leaf' and 'leave' or 'mat' and 'map' – and others being pairs of the same word. After saying each pair he will ask him to say whether the words are the same or different. He may also want him to write the words down. If a six year old makes five or more mistakes on a purely verbal twenty-pair test or, a seven year old makes four or more errors, then the psychologist will probably ask you to take your child for a special test to make sure there is nothing wrong with his hearing (see pages 85–6).

Tests for physical coordination

If during the preceding tests the psychologist notices that your child is not well coordinated, he may decide to carry out a systematic check on his overall physical coordination. The Oseretsky Tests are widely used around the world, and the ones I find give the most accurate results. They were developed by a Soviet psychologist of the same name in 1923, and were adapted for Western use by Robert H. Bruininks and are now known as the Bruininks-Oseretsky Tests of Motor Proficiency. They measure the maturity of your child's physical coordination by means of sets of six tasks which are graded according to age level. Each set consists of:

1. Body balancing while standing still.
2. A test for fine coordination using the hands to touch the tip of the nose with eyes closed, for example, or to trace through a maze.
3. A test of body-movement coordination – skipping, hopping or jumping.
4. A test of speed with both hands – threading beads or putting coins into a box.
5. Simultaneous movements with both hands, such as making circles in the air with index fingers extended and arms stretched out on either side.
6. Seeing how much one side of his body moves when carrying out a

task with the other side, such as clenching first one hand and then the other.

If your child cannot perform any one of the six tasks in the set for his age level, he will be tested on a set for a lower age level until he carries out all the tasks in a set correctly. Similarly, if he passes all the tests at his age level, he can attempt those intended for an older age group. The psychologist can then work out what is termed a 'motor age', which he can compare with your child's mental age, reading age and spelling age, which are known from the previous tests, as well as with his actual age.

The Oseretsky Tests take about a quarter of an hour to complete. The other test that is very commonly used is the Stott's Motor Impairment Test – a refinement of the Oseretsky Tests, which has been developed in Canada. If your child has great difficulty with these tests he might be referred for further investigations with a paediatric neurologist – a children's brain specialist.

We move on now to look at the tests which the psychologist may want your child to undergo elsewhere at a later date. These require equipment not normally available outside hospitals and specialist units. Obviously, the psychologist will delay his final diagnosis until he knows their results.

Tests that may be needed later

Eye tests
It is important your child's sight and vision are fully tested if the psychologist thinks it necessary. Most children will already have had their sight tested by having been asked to read letters of diminishing size from a chart across the room. This will have shown if they were nearsighted, because they would not have been able to see the letters clearly at a distance.

However, many parents are lulled into a false sense of security after this routine test, when they are told that their child's eyes are 'fine' – there are many other problems that can result in reading difficulties which this test will not reveal. For example, your child might be farsighted, being able to see distant objects clearly, but not those near to, such as letters in a book. Or there may be a fault in the way his two eyes converge for looking at things close up, which can put whatever he is concentrating on out of focus. If his eyes have been working in this way since birth, he will probably be unaware that what he is looking at is out of focus, because he has never seen anything sharply close to. For him blurred vision is normal, and he will think that everyone else sees in the same way.

Even when a child's focussing is less seriously affected, if his eyes do not converge perfectly on the page of the book he is trying to read, he will tend to read letters like 'p' and 'q' back to front, to read words with letters swopped round ('was' for 'saw'), to skip words in the line, lose his place or be unable to find the first word on the next line. If in addition he lacks smooth eye-muscle control, he will find it very hard to follow successive words in a line of print as his eyes sweep across the page. As a result of all these physical problems with his vision he will not understand what he reads and will give the impression that he is dyslexic (see Chapter 9).

If the psychologist who is carrying out the assessment suspects that your child's reading difficulties are a result of faulty vision, he will recommend you to make an appointment with an eye specialist – probably an orthoptist, or in the United States an optometrist, (someone who specializes in the coordination of eye movements) who has a particular interest in the way eyes develop throughout childhood. The orthoptist will check several aspects of your child's vision with various tests, including the Dunlop Test which shows whether he has a fixed reference eye for reading (see page 132), without which he will tend to read words with letters and syllables swopped round. In this particular test he will be asked to look at a picture down a machine called an amblyoscope, which has a separate tube for each eye. If the orthoptist's tests, which take in all about twenty minutes to perform, then confirm the psychologist's suspicions, he will refer your child to an ophthalmologist who will advise on the best way to rectify your child's vision, either with glasses or contact lenses, or with eye exercises or perhaps by patching one eye while reading (see page 132). Whatever type of treatment he prescribes, it is possible that it will greatly help your child with his reading difficulties.

Hearing test
If at the original assessment, the examiner thinks that your child's perception of spoken sounds is not as good as it should be, he will almost certainly refer you to a hospital or a centre with the sophisticated equipment necessary to carry out a hearing test. This is done to rule out the possibility of hearing loss which would affect his ability to identify high-frequency sounds such as /f/, /s/, /sh/, /th/ and /h/. This in turn would make it difficult for him to distinguish between words like 'thin' and 'fin', 'fat' and 'sat', 'gas' and 'gash', or 'this' and 'hiss'.

The test itself takes about half an hour. Your child will be given a pair of headphones to wear, through which will be played one at a time a random selection of tones at different frequencies – from very low to very high. He will simply be asked to say when he hears a tone. If he does not hear tones that come within the range of normal hearing, he will be referred to an ear specialist.

Depending on the extent of your child's hearing loss the specialist may prescribe a hearing aid or merely recommend him to sit at the front of the class. If the hearing loss is due to middle ear congestion – known as 'glue ears' – a minor operation may be necessary to drain the ear, after which tiny plastic tubes called grommets may be inserted in the ear-drum to allow continuous drainage until the problem is completely cleared up. The grommets can then be removed and the ear-drum will heal up again.

Test to discover his preferred ear

Just as most people are right- or left-handed and right- or left-eyed, so they are also right- or left-eared. The preferred ear for speech in non-dyslexics is usually the right, the preferred ear for non-verbal sounds, such as music or rustling leaves, being the left. The psychologist may want to know which your child's preferred ear is because it gives important clues about which side of his brain is most involved in dealing with language.

Most people are right-eared for speech and the messages from their right ear are interpreted by their brain's left hemisphere, which specialists now know to be the better half for processing language and ideas. Forty-five to sixty per cent of dyslexics, though, are left- or mixed-eared for speech, which means that more language than usual is being handled by the right hemisphere. This could account for reading and writing difficulties, because the right side of the brain is usually better at dealing with practical mechanical tasks like physical coordination, rather than logical ones such as constructing speech or interpreting letters or verbal sounds (see Chapter 9).

Again, the tests which might be used to find out your child's preferred ear – termed 'dichotic listening tasks' – require special equipment, so if the psychologist thinks they are necessary, he will refer you to an appropriate clinic. Despite its grand-sounding name, the procedures used in dichotic listening will be easy for your child to follow. He will be given a pair of stereo headphones to put on. Into one ear will be played a recording of a voice saying random groups of three numbers – '1,9,5', then, '3,1,7', and so on. Simultaneously into his other ear will be played the same voice at the same volume saying different groups of three numbers – '2,4,9', then, '6,5,8', for example. After each set of numbers has been played, he will be asked to say out loud what he has heard. He will tend to report the numbers he has heard in his preferred ear for speech more often than the ones heard in the other ear.

As I said at the beginning of the chapter, this is not an exhaustive list of all the tests your child might be given, but it does cover the ones most commonly used. Once the psychologist has the results of any specialist examinations he may have requested you to attend after his initial assessment, he can compare them with his own findings and arrive at a diagnosis, which should include a full description of the type of teaching needed and the areas of difficulty your child is experiencing, with suggestions for overcoming them. If your child is indeed dyslexic, then your first priority should be to make every effort to see that he gets some form of specialist remedial teaching for his problem. And it is to this subject that I now want to turn.

7. HOW SUCCESSFUL IS SPECIALIST TEACHING?

Who gives it?

I have already described in Chapter 4 the ways in which parents and schools should try to ensure that a diagnosed dyslexic child receives specialist remedial teaching. To recap briefly here, there are four main avenues of approach.

1. Many schools, both private and State maintained, will now allow specialist teachers (resource teachers in Australia) to come into school and give lessons to those children who are having difficulties with reading and writing.
2. Depending on where you live, the local education authority might be able to arrange for your child to attend a specialist dyslexia clinic or centre.
3. There may be a teacher qualified in dyslexic teaching among the school staff. (This is the most likely course in the United States.)
4. You can arrange for private tutoring by a specialist teacher who has been recommended either by the psychologist or school counsellor who diagnosed your child, your family doctor, your local dyslexia association (see Appendix for addresses), your child's school or even friends with dyslexic children.

There are pros and cons to each of the above. If your child is given specialist tutoring in school, he will benefit from not missing too much school time, and sessions can be scheduled at times when his school work is least disrupted. On the other hand, if he has lessons at a specialist centre, this may give you, his parents, the opportunity to accompany him and become actively involved in the therapy. Where this is possible, I have found that children usually make much better progress. Also, your child will be learning to read and write in a setting where his disability does not set him apart from his fellow pupils. One tip when organizing times for classes outside school hours is not to make them clash with other activities your child is looking forward to, otherwise he will resent remedial help and look on his extra lessons merely as a chore.

There is, officially, no such professional as a 'dyslexia therapist'. Specialist teachers will be, for example, speech therapists, psychologists or schoolteachers who have an extra qualification in dyslexic teaching. So if you are planning on private tutoring, it is essential to find out where the specialist teacher was trained, for how long and what their track record is like. Local dyslexia associations and psychologists in the field should be able to provide all the necessary information.

What exactly does specialist teaching do?

Obviously, one particular method of specialist teaching will not suit every single dyslexic child, so teachers and therapists need to have a number of techniques at their fingertips to be able to meet every failing reader's needs. However, phonetic/linguistic tutoring along the carefully structured lines I described for schoolteachers in Chapter 5 has proved effective in virtually all centres where it is used for teaching dyslexic children.

This type of dyslexia-oriented therapy does not assume the child knows anything unless it has been specifically taught, and in this way is rather like teaching language to a foreigner. Even when he shows some understanding of reading and spelling, the specialist has to check from the beginning to make sure there are no gaps in his knowledge which will create a shaky foundation to build on. It is not just a way of taking the dyslexic more slowly along the road to literacy, but of providing a very logical, systematic and thorough road where everything makes sense, so that his alert mind can grasp the logic and make use of it.

The usual methods of teaching reading and spelling in school (see pages 58–60), which are perfectly satisfactory for the majority of children, do not work for the dyslexic, and there is no way he can learn to spell from lists of words with unrelated spelling patterns. He may remember a few for a test next day, but will certainly not retain their spelling in his memory for longer, unless he has a good grounding in phonetics – the way single letters and combinations of letters sound – to give him some clues.

Phonetic/linguistic therapy aims to give him that grounding. It teaches him the techniques of spelling that most other people simply take for granted. For example, I don't suppose that you have given much thought to the fact that the letter 'c' is pronounced /s/ when it is followed by an 'e', 'i' or 'y' as in 'city', 'century' or 'cygnet'. You have not thought about it because you don't have to, you have picked it up naturally without having to analyse it. But this principle needs to be explained to the dyslexic. This may seem overcomplicated, but for the dyslexic, reading and spelling do not just 'happen', they have to be taught scientifically, with every step of the way clarified and made comprehensible.

In addition to specially geared reading and writing tuition, specialist dyslexia therapy should also give help, when needed, with mathematics, directional confusion, telling the time and all the other typical problem areas for the dyslexic.

How effective is specialist teaching?

In a study carried out in 1978 at Bangor University in north Wales, Prof Tim Miles and I found that the dyslexia-oriented therapy provided in three specialist centres was more effective than the teaching given in standard remedial reading and writing classes in schools, which is not aimed specifically at dyslexics but at all bad readers, including those with low IQs. In the dyslexia centres, the average gain in pupils' reading and spelling skills was two years for every year of treatment. Before treatment, the children had been slipping behind from the beginning of their schooling and were on average two to two and a half years behind in their literary ability. These results suggest that most dyslexics would need around two years of this sort of teaching to bring them up to an acceptable level. Once they have reached it, they generally do not slip back and so do not need further specialist teaching, although it may help to have short refresher courses before important exams. Of course, this is a broad generalization which won't apply to everyone, but it gives you a rough idea of the time-scale involved.

The effect that specialist phonetic/linguistic teaching has on dyslexic children can best be illustrated by showing the sort of progress that can be made. This I have done by including the following four case histories of pupils whose dyslexia was successfully treated at our clinic at St Bartholomew's Hospital in London. Not every child will respond as well as these did, but it is seldom that little or no progress is made unless there are very definite reasons.

Four success stories

I have chosen to show the advances made by these particular four children because by and large they represent the broad spectrum of dyslexia. Although each one has a different type of dyslexia, they all responded well to the structured, multisensory, phonetic/linguistic method of specialist teaching. I hope parents of recently diagnosed dyslexic children will take heart from these case histories. As you will see, at the time of their assessments these children's writing and spelling seemed almost beyond hope, yet by the end of their remedial programmes all had made remarkable strides and were able to produce acceptable written work.

Before reading these case histories I would advise you to read through the diagnostic tests described in the previous chapter if you decided to skip them. I shall be mentioning in detail the results of the tests we performed on these children, because this is the best way to give you the clearest possible picture of their dyslexia.

Denis: uninherited or acquired dyslexia
His background Denis came from a highly literate family – his mother

and father were both university lecturers – which had no truly positive history of reading and spelling difficulties. It seems that his dyslexia resulted either from minor maldevelopment in the womb or from slight damage to his brain at the time of birth. He was twelve days overdue and the labour was very long. Denis was a large baby, over 10 lb (4.5 kg), with a large head, but as nothing abnormal was found he and his mother returned from hospital after two weeks. All his faculties developed normally, except speech which was very late. Even by the age of four, he was only able to manage single syllables – such as /bŏ/ for 'bottle'.

When he started State school at five, his speech was still completely unintelligible; he was, of course, unable to read or write; and being very clumsy, was rejected by the other children because he spoiled their games. Denis became desperately unhappy and cried every morning before going to school. Eventually he developed a school phobia, getting frequent headaches and stomach-aches which enabled him to stay at home.

At six he was referred to a child psychiatrist because of his learning difficulties and his increasingly aggressive behaviour. A year later he saw a paediatrician – a doctor who specializes in childhood illnesses – who told his parents that he was a clumsy child, but advised them not to worry, as he would grow out of it.

Diagnosis At the age of ten, and still unable to read, Denis eventually came to the Dyslexia Clinic at St Bartholomew's Hospital. Our assessment revealed that he was undoubtedly dyslexic.

Denis was a crossed lateral (see page 81) – in other words was left-handed but right-eyed – which meant that he had innate problems following a line of print from left to right. He was left-eared for verbal sounds, which suggested that his language area was not fully sited in the left hemisphere of his brain — the better half for dealing with words and ideas (see pages 126–9). His pencil control was poor and he was unable to manage the three-fingered grip that most people use. His movements were jerky and he was constantly knocking things over and tripping over things. His class teacher reckoned that he was unable to learn because he spent most of his time picking his belongings up off the floor! He was extremely sensitive to loud aggressive voices, which made him totally unresponsive to teachers who habitually shouted at him.

Denis could not tell the time and his general concept of time was very poor. But he was obsessive about it, since he could never work out in advance how long anything would take to accomplish. He also had terrible problems with dressing himself, always putting shoes on the wrong feet, clothes on back to front, buttons in the wrong holes, and having his tie and shoe-laces undone or askew. He had great difficulty in copying anything from the board or even from a book.

His speech was still not up to the level expected of a ten year old. When asked to describe something verbally his answers were long-winded and formless. He found it very hard to get his thoughts and ideas into any proper order, and would punctuate his talk with such remarks as, 'Where was I?', and, 'What was I talking about just now?' He had other sequencing problems as well, such as being unable to recite the alphabet, the months of the year, multiplication tables or the usual order of daily events.

His IQ was assessed by testing him on the Wechsler Intelligence Scale for Children (WISC), which is described in detail in the previous chapter. His scores placed him in the average range of intelligence and there was no significant difference between his verbal and non-verbal, or performance, ability, both being within the Normal range.

Verbal tests	Scaled score out of 20 (Average 10)
Information	13
Comprehension	10
Arithmetic	9
Similarities	12
Vocabulary	13
(Digit span)	(5)

Performance tests	Scaled score out of 20 (Average 10)
Picture completion	10
Picture arrangement	10
Block design	10
Object assembly	11
Coding	3

Verbal IQ	109	⎫
Performance IQ	92	⎬ Average 100
Full-scale IQ	101	⎭

Other tests revealed that he was two years behind his age in physical coordination and that he lagged by over four years in perception of verbal sounds, shape-copying, and reading and spelling. You can see in *Fig 1* his effort at the Midland Spelling Test (see also page 80). He managed to spell

Fig 1

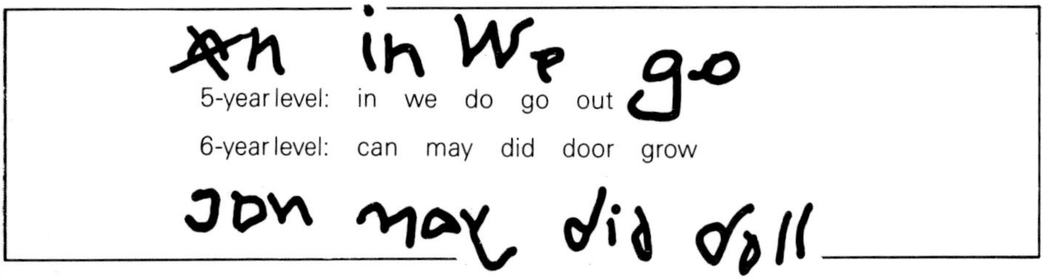

5-year level: in we do go out

6-year level: can may did door grow

91

Figs 2a & b

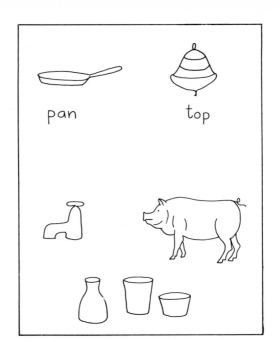

What Denis's teacher drew on the board for the class to copy.

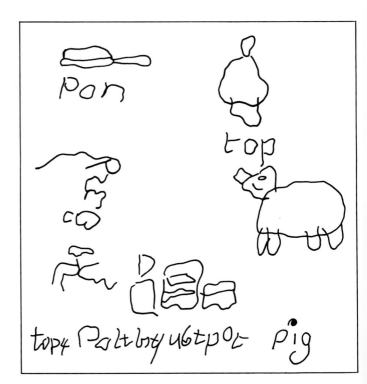

Denis's effort at copying his teacher's model.

correctly three words that were read out to him from the line which a normal five year old should be able to cope with, but could only manage 'did', 'can' and 'may' from the six-year-old level, the 'c' in 'can' and the 'y' in 'may' being mirror written.

His progress through our programme *Fig 2* is a sample of the work Denis was doing at school just before he came to the clinic for treatment. He was trying to copy what the teacher had drawn and written on the board – further evidence of his difficulty not only with written words, but also with copying shapes.

The next example (*Fig 3*) also comes from his school work before he began special therapy. He was trying to copy some work which his teacher had written out for him. It was meant to be a diary of what he had done the day before – work which the other children were writing up on their own. It reads:

Tuesday
Today we watched television and . . . .

Fig 3

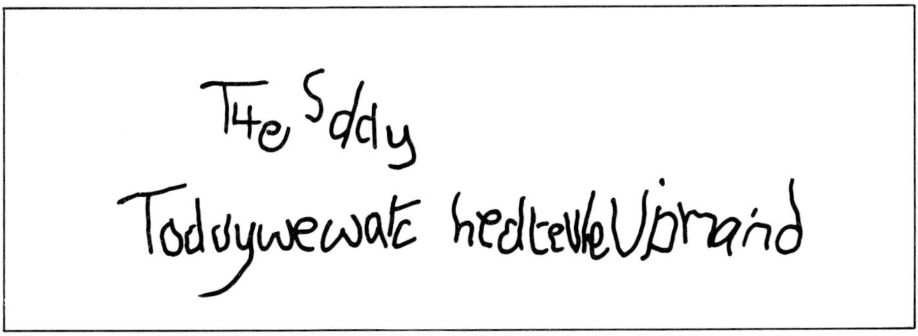

Denis gave up after that. It is clear that he had no idea what he was writing, could not read it and did not understand that written words have to have a gap between them to show where one word ends and the next begins.

Fig 4 was written after six months' treatment. Denis was amazed to discover that there was a relationship between the sounds in words and

Fig 4

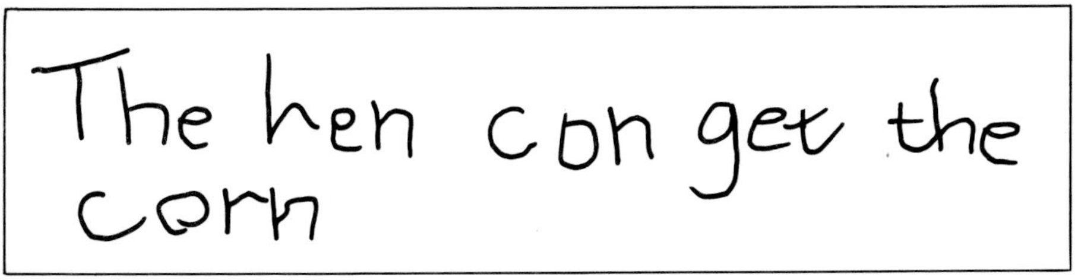

the shapes you put down on paper. Up until then he had assumed it was just guesswork and that he must be a terrible guesser. You can see that he is still mirror writing the letter 'a', but is definitely latching onto the idea that words have sound patterns, and is beginning to gain confidence by writing simple words intelligibly.

By *Fig 5* he is around eighteen months into his treatment and is progressing steadily through the remedial programme, learning the first of the silent-letter rules: namely, if there is a silent letter before an 'n' it will be a 'k' or a 'g'. Here he is practising silent 'k'. In the free writing of Fig 5 he has not yet mastered joining up the letters but his handwriting is vastly improved. In the word 'knight' he has mixed up the spelling pattern of the final 'e', lengthening the preceding vowel with the 'igh' pattern which produces a long vowel anyway without adding an 'e'. And he nearly forgot the silent 'k' in the word 'knife' but these are the only careless spelling mistakes – you can see from the rest of the passage that he understands the spelling patterns which govern those two words. Denis has now learnt about punctuation, and can use full stops, commas, quotation marks

Fig 5

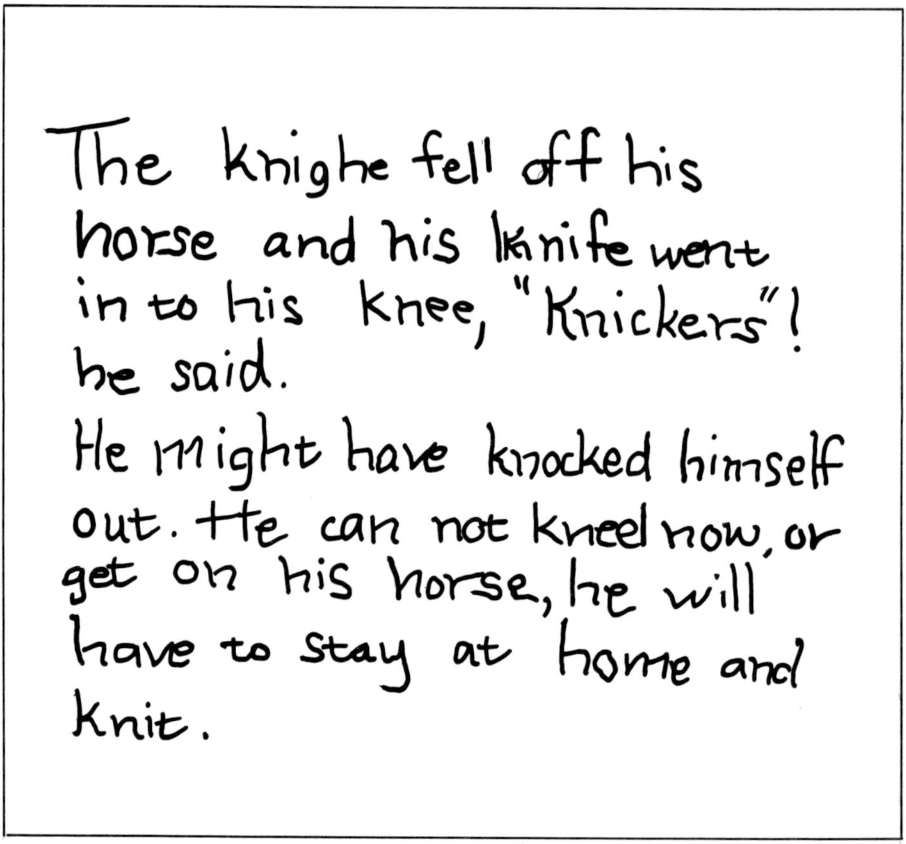

The knighe fell off his horse and his knife went in to his knee, "Knickers"! he said.
He might have knocked himself out. He can not kneel now, or get on his horse, he will have to stay at home and knit.

and exclamation marks, and also knows where to make paragraphs and when to use capital letters. Note also the touches of humour that he now brings to his writing, which give an insight into his change of attitude, not only to his disability, but also to life in general. He is beginning to do very well at school and enjoys every moment – even gymnastics at which he used to be very bad. He became particularly good at trampolining.

The free writing in *Fig 6* was produced at the age of twelve and a half, after two and a half years' specialist therapy. Denis's handwriting is now becoming much smaller and neater, and his spelling more sophisticated. He still occasionally adds or omits a letter, but that is all. At this stage in the programme we are learning that words of Greek origin have 'ph' to represent the /f/ sound – as in 'triumph' in the first line. Denis can read virtually anything by this stage.

The passage in *Fig 7* was written four years after he first came to our clinic and is an excerpt from a very long essay produced for his school about the First World War. He used a very original format, writing it as a letter from one German soldier to another. Denis had recently finished

Fig 6

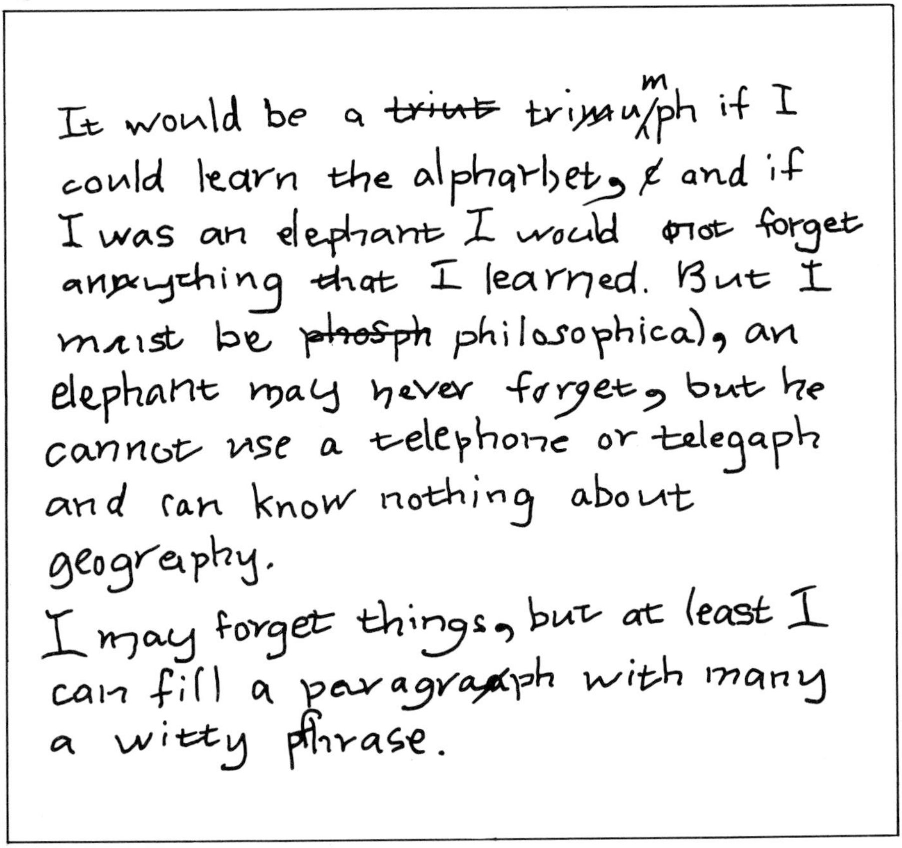

It would be a ~~triut~~ triu^m/ph if I could learn the alpharbet, ¢ and if I was an elephant I would ~~not~~ forget any~~thing~~ that I learned. But I maist be ~~phosph~~ philosophical, an elephant may never forget, but he cannot use a telephone or telegaph and can know nothing about geography.
I may forget things, but at least I can fill a paragra~~a~~ph with many a witty phrase.

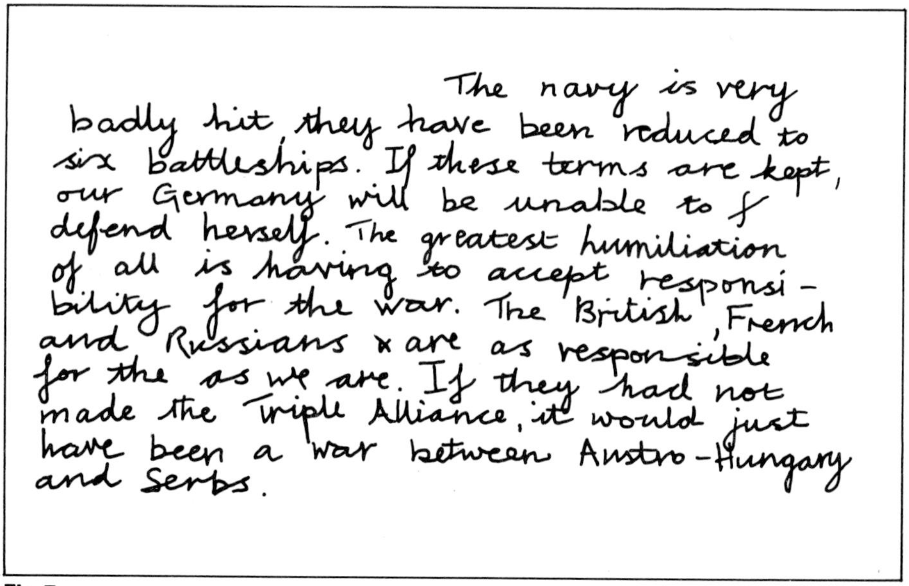

> The navy is very badly hit, they have been reduced to six battleships. If these terms are kept, our Germany will be unable to f defend herself. The greatest humiliation of all is having to accept responsibility for the war. The British, French and Russians x are as responsible for the as we are. If they had not made the Triple Alliance, it would just have been a war between Austro-Hungary and Serbs.

Fig 7

his therapy but brought the essay in to show me, as he had received 10 out of 10 for it and it had been judged the best in the class. He had been asked to read it out aloud and had been greatly praised. Needless to say, he was extremely pleased, and it was a marvellous achievement in view of the severity of his original condition. This seemed to be the turning point in his realization that he had a good brain which he was now determined to use to the full.

It was clear that he was a far more intelligent boy than was at first realized. At the age of fifteen we decided to reassess his intelligence and found that in five years his full-scale IQ had risen from 101 to 130, placing him in the Very Superior range of intelligence along with the top 2.2 per cent of the population. It is very unusual for IQs to change by more than a few points as children grow older, and in Denis's case we could only assume that his emotional problems early on had held up his intellectual development.

The outcome At the age of sixteen, two years after he finished his remedial programme, Denis passed his first public exams in the following subjects: English, English Language, Spoken English, Geography, History, Biology, Chemistry, Mathematics and Social Studies. Two years later he passed pre-college exams in economics and geography, and at the time of writing is studying for a degree in geography.

The examples you have seen of his writing and spelling show clearly that specialist teaching worked dramatically well for Denis. But I am convinced that had he been sent to us at an earlier age, he would have made faster progress and an even more complete recovery.

96

Thomas: typical inherited dyslexia

His background   Thomas came from a working-class family living in the East End of London. Several of his close relatives had been late learning to read and were still bad spellers, and some were also left-handed. Thomas's birth and the preceding pregnancy were normal, and the only skill he was late in developing as a toddler was talking. He was five before he said anything, and even then only his mother could understand him. His speech improved of its own accord without speech therapy, so that by the time he first came to the Bart's Clinic the only problems which remained were that he sometimes could not put a name to an object or person, and occasionally used incorrect words in conversation, such as, 'English competition', instead of, 'English composition'.

Diagnosis   Thomas was referred to the clinic by his State school because of his lack of progress with reading, writing and spelling, and I gave him an assessment three months before his thirteenth birthday. His scores on the WISC intelligence test (described in detail in the previous chapter) showed that he was in the Top Average intelligence range, with no real imbalance between his verbal and non-verbal abilities.

Verbal tests	Scaled score out of 20 (Average 10)
Information	8
Comprehension	17
Arithmetic	10
Similarities	15
Vocabulary	10
(Digit span)	(8)

Performance tests	Scaled score out of 20 (Average 10)
Picture completion	12
Picture arrangement	10
Block design	10
Object assembly	12
Coding	8

Verbal IQ	113	
Performance IQ	103	Average 100
Full-scale IQ	109	

We discovered that Thomas was behind by over four years in reading and by five years in his spelling. Other tests showed that he could only distinguish between similar-sounding spoken words with the competence of a

Figs 8a & b

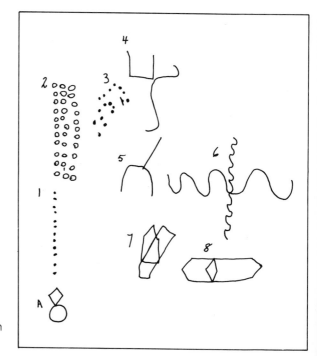

The Bender-Gestalt shape-copying test. All the shapes are presented on separate cards—not together on one sheet as shown here.

Thomas's attempt at the Bender-Gestalt test. Note that the relationships between the items are not important, as he was shown each one separately.

seven year old and was at a six and a half year old's level when copying shapes (see *Fig 8*).

We also found that he was a crossed lateral, being right-handed but left-eyed (see page 81). He was unsure of the order of the alphabet, he left out some months of the year, was unable to recite multiplication tables, and muddled up syllables in long words.

Thomas was exceptionally tall for his age, but otherwise there was nothing unusual about him physically or emotionally. He came across as very thoughtful and cheerful with a good sense of humour and was well coordinated – in fact he was an excellent athlete. Unlike Denis in the previous case history, Thomas's dyslexia did not seem to have affected his emotional well-being.

The examples of his work that follow are considerably better than Denis's, as Thomas was two years older and his spelling age was two and a half years more advanced. However, they do show a marked improvement from the start of specialist treatment to the end.

His progress through our programme   *Fig 8* shows Thomas's assessment attempt at the Bender-Gestalt shape-copying test (see also page 83). Although he was nearly thirteen, this effort only reached the level you would expect from a six and a half year old. He has drawn items A, 1 and 2 downwards instead of across the page. Item 3 has lost its form, while 5 is composed of continuous lines rather than dots. There are far too many wiggles in 6, and he has flattened the ends of both overlapping shapes in 7.

Thomas wrote the sentences in *Fig 9* at the beginning of his treatment. His handwriting is very immature – he had originally been taught 'ball-and-stick' letters (see also page 69) which he had been unable to convert into joined-up writing. The capital 'T' in the word 'Tom' is written like a capital 'J' and he always used a capital 'J' when it should have been a

Fig 9

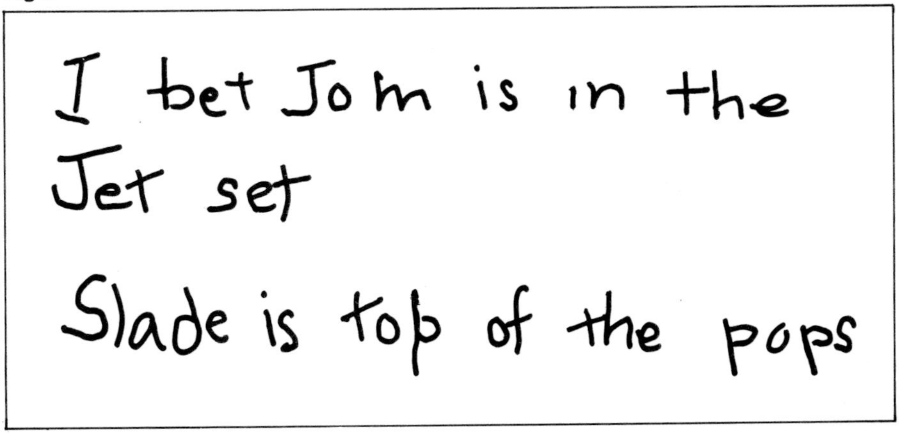

I bet Jo m is in the
Jet set

Slade is top of the pops

little 'j', as in 'Jet'. He not only shows traces of 'b'/'d' confusion in the shape of the 'b' in 'bet', but you can also see that he has trouble distinguishing between 'b' and 'p', as in the word 'top'.

The writing in *Fig 10* was produced after two months' remedial tuition. Thomas is trying hard to add linking strokes to his letters and manages them with the 't' in 'tank', the 'a' in 'was' and the 'e' in 'very'. However, the habit of using 'ball-and-stick' letters is deeply engrained by this age and was proving very hard to overcome. He is still showing confusion between 'd' and 'g' in the last letter of 'bang'. At this stage of the programme he is learning how the sound of 'n' changes when it is paired with 'g' and 'k', as in 'tank' and 'bang'.

Fig 10

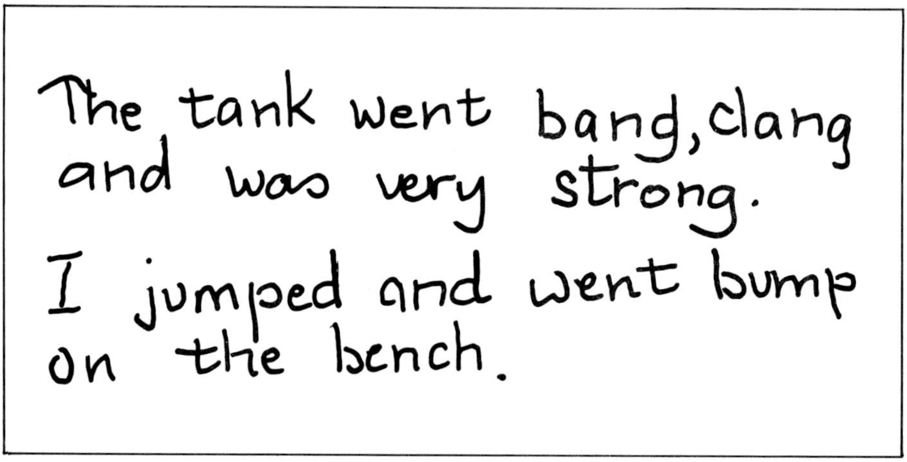

The tank went bang, clang
and was very strong.
I jumped and went bump
on the bench.

The sentences in *Fig 11* are taken from work done nine months into the remedial programme. Thomas's letter forms are now more controlled and he is much better at keeping his writing in a straight line. At this point he is practising changing the sound of words ending in /ar/ by adding an 'e' on the end.

Fig 11

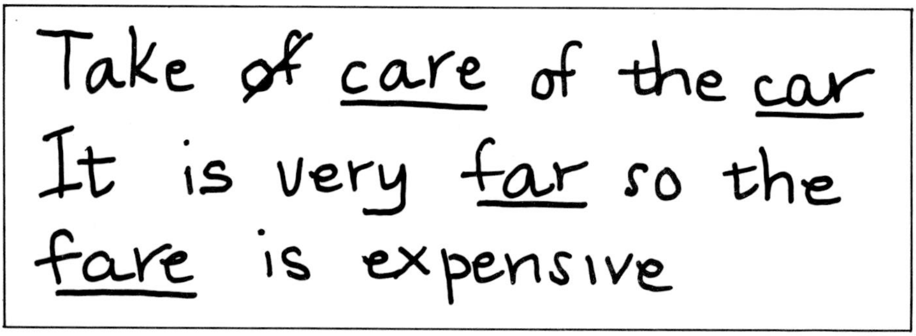

Take of care of the car
It is very far so the
fare is expensive

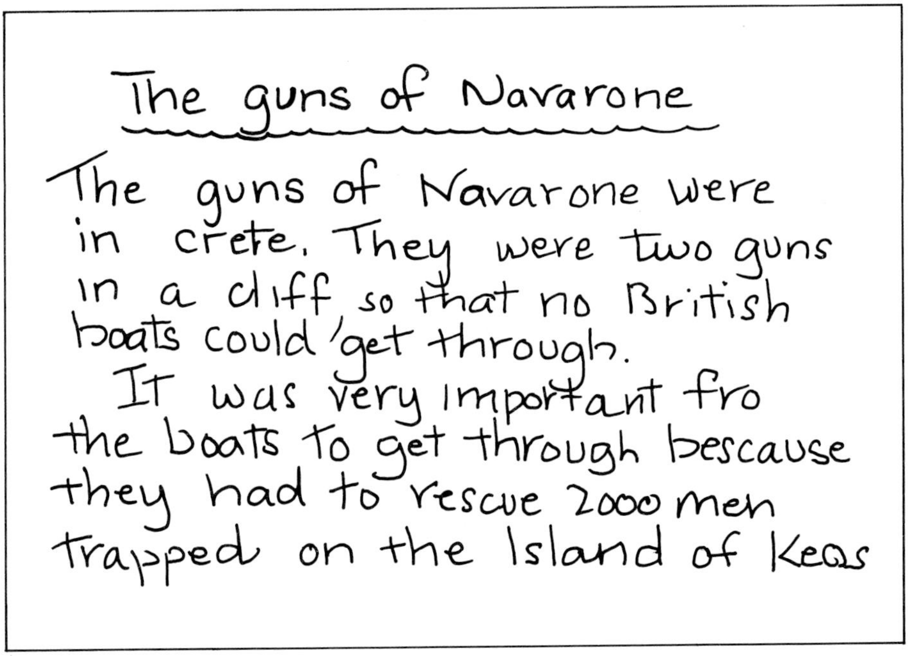

The guns of Navarone

The guns of Navarone were in crete. They were two guns in a cliff so that no British boats could get through.
It was very important fro the boats to get through bescause they had to rescue 2000 men trapped on the Island of Keos

Fig 12

The outcome The final example, *Fig 12*, was written a year and a half after *Fig 11*. Thomas has now progressed to essay writing, but unfortunately has had to give up trying to join up the letters. The change to joined-up writing was making his work too untidy. He continued to make occasional dyslexic mistakes, such as 'fro' for 'for' in line 5, and 'bescause' in line 6. But overall Thomas made excellent progress and his performance at school surpassed everyone's expectations. Soon after he finished his two-year course at St Bartholomew's I received a letter from Thomas's mother which read:

> Thomas has had an excellent report and we are very pleased with him. We were delighted to find out that he has earned this year's form prize for the highest overall exam marks. He is taking it all very calmly but we have given him lots of pats on the back. We are amazed at the confidence he has built up over the last two years. He is enjoying his selected subjects and is working well.

This was exciting news, but once again, as with Denis, if we had been able to give Thomas appropriate teaching at a much earlier age, I am sure we would have been able to iron out most of the remaining problems with his spelling. His future might well have been even brighter than it is now.

Janice: low verbal ability but good visual skills

Her background Janice came from a middle-class family with a strong history of dyslexia, many of them being left-handed. All went well at Janice's birth, so the evidence points to her condition being inherited.

Like the boys in the previous two case histories, Denis and Thomas, she was a very late talker – as her mother said, when speech did begin to emerge, 'She might have been talking Chinese.' And she made no progress with reading or writing at school. At the age of six she was seen by a psychologist who did not diagnose dyslexia. Janice was not a trouble-maker, so there was no objection to her continuing at her State school, where she sat at the back of the class and took hardly any part in lessons. Not surprisingly, she learnt little over the next five years.

Diagnosis At eight and a half she was eventually diagnosed alexic – that is, totally unable to read or write – by specialists at London's National Hospital for Nervous Diseases. There she was given the WISC intelligence test (described in the previous chapter) and her results were as follows:

Verbal tests	Scaled score out of 20 (Average 10)
Information	4
Arithmetic	5
Similarities	6
Vocabulary	11
(Digit span)	(6)

Performance tests	Scaled score out of 20 (Average 10)
Picture completion	14
Picture arrangement	15
Block design	15

Verbal IQ	81 (prorated)	
Performance IQ	131 (estimated)	Average 100
Full-scale IQ	105	

The big difference between verbal and performance IQs is a common sign that a child will have some kind of learning difficulty, but her high performance IQ suggested that she would be good at practical tasks. In spite of Janice's good visual skills she was not able to learn to read at school by the whole-word 'Look and Say' method (see page 59). She was given no effective remedial help by her local education authority and soon after she turned eleven was eventually referred to us at St Bartholomew's.

At that time she had a reading age of a seven year old and her spelling was so bad when tested that we were unable to give it a score. Her reading and writing difficulties were more severe than those of the children mentioned so far in this chapter. We found that Janice was right-handed and left-eyed – a crossed lateral, and was also strongly left-eared (see page 81). This meant that not only did she have trouble following a line of print from left to right, but also that more language than normal was being processed in the right-hand side of her brain – the side better suited to handling spatial and visual tasks. Although she had no actual speech defects at the time of her assessment, she was extremely slow at understanding language and grasping new ideas.

When she began treatment she could not write a word – except for her first name, nor could she write out the alphabet, nor recite the months of the year. She could not tell the time, and her concept of time and space was extremely muddled. Even by the age of thirteen she could not tell what day of the week it was, when Christmas was, or what time she might be expected to go to bed.

Although she found it very hard to distinguish between words that sounded alike when spoken, she was still able to learn by the phonetically structured method, which relies largely on being taught how letters sound both singly and in groups (see Chapter 5). Indeed, this was the only way that written language made sense to her. Janice attended the clinic for three years, and although progress was slow and hard, she did achieve a very acceptable level of reading and writing. When you see her early efforts, you can understand why her parents believed at the time that recovery was impossible.

Her progress through our programme   When asked at her assessment to spell the easiest five words of the spelling test – 'see', 'cut', 'mat', 'in' and 'ran', Janice only managed to write down:

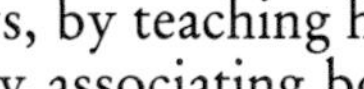

I then dictated the alphabet to see if she knew the shapes of the letters and she produced the first eleven letters as in *Fig 13*. They are neat and well formed, but she was unable to string them together to make a word. All she could write from memory was her first name.

We began, as always, by teaching her the names of the letters, the sounds they represent, and by associating both of these concepts to the shapes of the letters. From there we began to build simple words, such as 'cap',

Fig 13

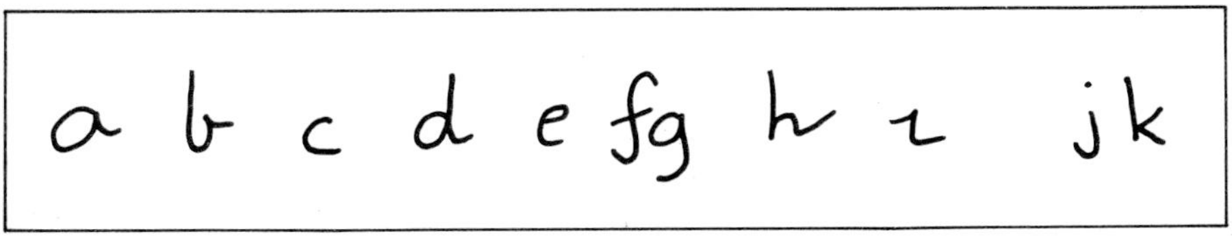

'wet', 'not', and so on. Once these had been learnt, we began to construct simple sentences such as, 'The cat wet the bed', or, 'The sun is hot.' Gradually more spelling patterns were introduced such as the blending of consonants in words like 'flash' and 'grab', and the lengthening of a vowel by adding 'e' to the end of a word – as in 'hat' and 'hate'.

The sentences in *Fig 14* were written after eighteen months of specialist tutoring. At this stage Janice is being taught that certain combinations of vowels produce only one sound, as in words like 'sail' and 'boat'. In this particular exercise she is learning that the long /ō/ sound in these words will either be spelt 'oa', if the sound is at the beginning or in the middle of the word – as in 'loaf' – or 'ow', if the sound comes at the end of a word – as in 'mow'. She has picked up this idea very well and has developed good clear joined-up writing.

Fig 14

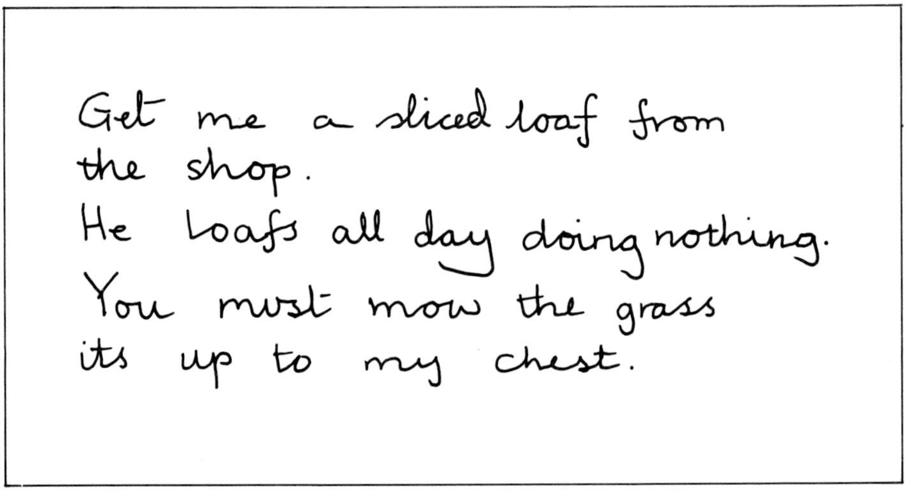

> Get me a sliced loaf from the shop.
> He loafs all day doing nothing.
> You must mow the grass its up to my chest.

In *Fig 15*, written a few months later, Janice is being taught that the spelling 'oo' can have either a long sound, as in the word 'fōod', or a short sound, as in 'bŏok'.

Fig 15

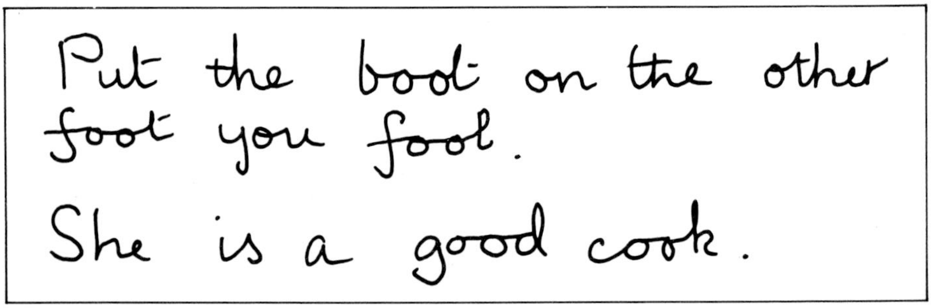

> Put the boot on the other foot you fool.
> She is a good cook.

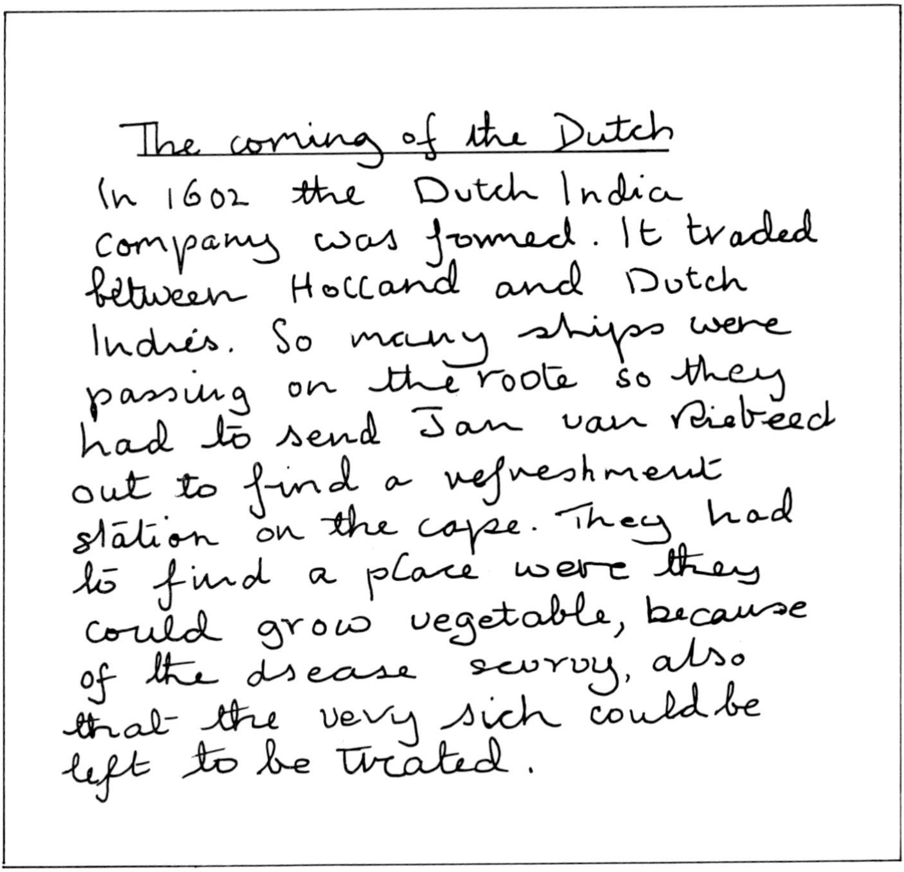

The coming of the Dutch

In 1602 the Dutch India company was formed. It traded between Holland and Dutch Indies. So many ships were passing on the roote so they had to send Jan van Riebeed out to find a refreshment station on the cape. They had to find a place were they could grow vegetable, because of the dsease scurvy, also that the very sich could be left to be treated.

Fig 16

After nearly three years on our programme, Janice was able to write a very commendable essay, and *Fig 16* is the first paragraph of a piece of school work which won her the class teacher's unreserved praise. She is tending to write rather fast here and is therefore less neat than she used to be, but her thoughts can flow much better when she writes this way. Even so, she does make occasional spelling mistakes – 'dsease' in the third line up from the bottom, and 'route' spelled 'roote' in the fifth line, for instance – but they are very minor and do not in any way affect the meaning of the passage.

The outcome Janice continued into the pre-college class where she matured greatly. She passed her first public exams at the age of sixteen in English, Mathematics, Science, History, Geography, Art and Crafts, Technical Drawing and Domestic Science. She received an excellent final report from her school, who stressed the fact that she was an extremely hard-working, responsible and likeable girl who deserved to do well in life.

When Janice left school she was offered a place at a catering college but decided to learn 'the hard way'. She has been working in the kitchen of a restaurant for over a year now and reckons she has learnt as much about cooking as she would ever have done at college. Having watched her diligent struggle to overcome her dyslexia pay off, I have no doubt that she will eventually find her niche in life and make a great success of it.

Henry: a bright dyslexic discovered early

His background   At the age of five Henry was given speech therapy for slow language development and a mild speech defect. Although he understood everything that was said to him, he was one and a half years behind in his expressive language, and had difficulty pronouncing /l/, /r/, /th/ and /y/. After a year's therapy his speech was restored to normal.

Soon afterwards, though, at the age of six, his father, an international lawyer, was asked to remove him from his private school because he was unable to read. As so many children with early speech and language difficulties have continuing problems with written language, his speech therapist suggested that he might be dyslexic.

Diagnosis   These suspicions were borne out at his assessment at St Bartholomew's Dyslexia Clinic. We discovered that several members of Henry's family were late readers and poor spellers, although none seemed to have had early speech defects or were left-handed. There had been no complications at his birth and apart from his speech, all his other abilities, such as walking, had developed normally into toddlerhood.

His intelligence was measured on the WISC test (described in the previous chapter) and the results were as follows:

Verbal tests	Scaled score out of 20 (Average 10)
Information	19
Comprehension	20
Arithmetic	13
Similarities	19
Vocabulary	18
(Digit span)	(8)

Performance tests	Scaled score out of 20 (Average 10)
Picture completion	14
Picture arrangement	14
Block design	14
Object assembly	15
Coding	8

Verbal IQ	149 ⎫	
Performance IQ	121 ⎬	Average 100
Full-scale IQ	139 ⎭	

This is an extremely high score that places Henry in the Very Superior range of intelligence, in company with the top 2.2 per cent of the population. His relatively lower performance IQ suggested that he would do better in arts subjects rather than in mathematics or sciences. His low scores on the Digit Span and Coding tests showed up typical dyslexic sequencing difficulties.

He scored nil in his reading and spelling tests. I cannot show an example of Henry's work written before starting treatment, since he could not read or write anything at all – not even his name.

His progress through our programme We had to begin, of course, by teaching him the letters of the alphabet, their shapes and sounds. He was quick on the uptake and made rapid progress. Six months later he wrote the sentences in *Fig 17*. Although the letters are a little shaky and he has spelt 'got' as 'god', this is an amazing leap forward. He has made few mistakes and is already managing to join up his letters without them looking too untidy. He sometimes repeats words or phrases – 'at the' appearing twice in the same sentence.

Fig 17

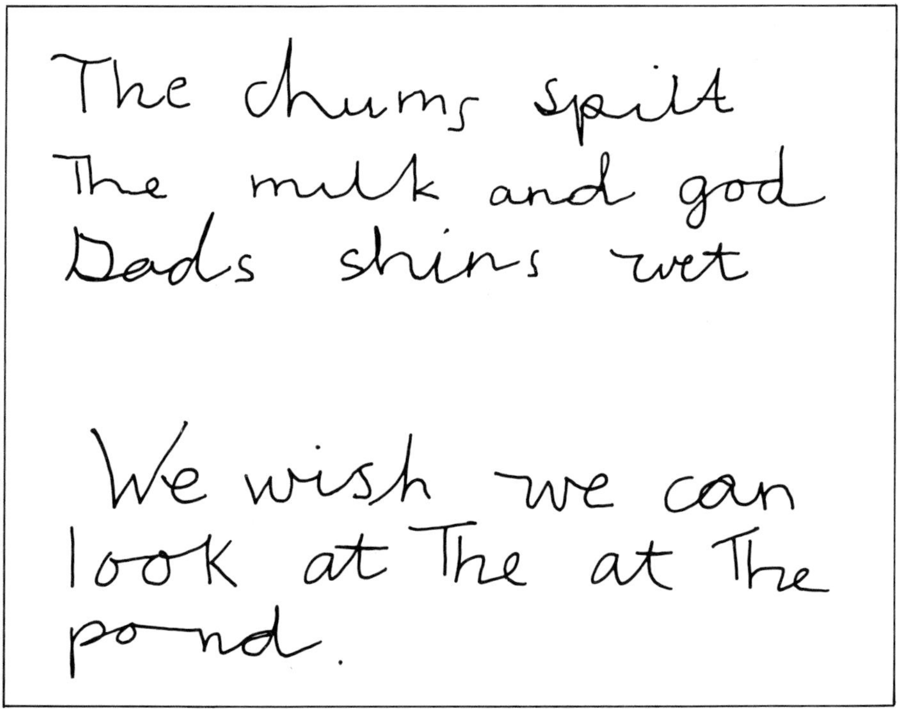

The chums spilt
The milk and god
Dads shins wet

We wish we can
look at The at The
pond.

He cut her frowt
Puff the pipe nine times

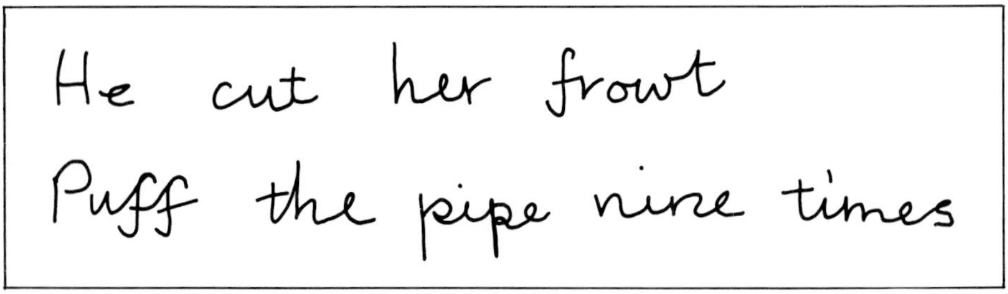

Fig 18

Six months later, a year into the programme, his handwriting in *Fig 18* is now more controlled and flowing, and he has learnt more complicated spelling patterns, such as the combination 'er' in 'her', and the 'i' in 'pipe' sounding long because of the final 'e'. Note that his earlier speech problem of mixing up /f/ and /th/ now occasionally surfaces in his spelling too – 'frowt' for 'throat'.

After two years in treatment, at the age of 8 years 3 months, Henry had achieved an accuracy reading age of 9 years 5 months, and a comprehension reading age of 11 years 2 months. His spelling had improved to 8 years 8 months – just above his real age. These are excellent results, but are what a dyslexia specialist would be hoping for, considering his very high IQ.

His free writing at that time (see *Fig 19*) indicates that his interest in history was already showing itself. There are several errors here that will be obvious to any good speller, but it is a well-sustained piece of creative prose for such a young dyslexic.

Fig 19

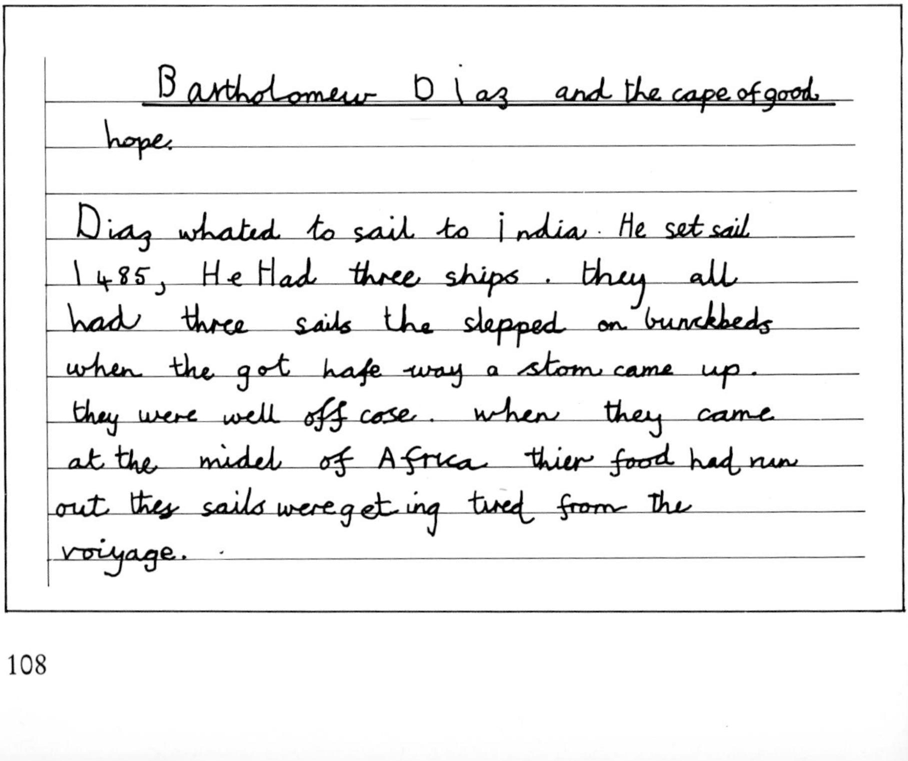

Barthalomew D i az and the cape of good
hope.

Diaz whated to sail to india. He set sail
1485, He Had three ships. they all
had three sails the slepped on bunckbeds
when the got hafe way a stom came up.
they were well off cose. when they came
at the midel of Africa thier food had run
out they sails weregeting tired from the
voiyage.

Three months later, shortly before his treatment was finished, he wrote a first-class essay about a town in Roman Britain. You can see the first few lines in *Fig 20*. By now nearly all his spelling mistakes are gone.

Fig 20

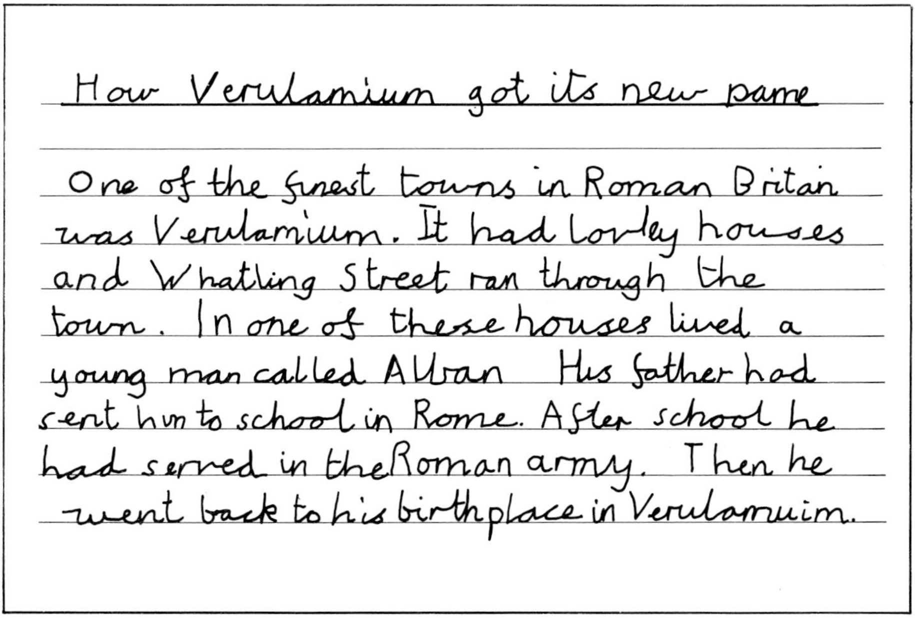

> How Verulamium got its new name
>
> One of the finest towns in Roman Britain was Verulamium. It had lovely houses and Whatling Street ran through the town. In one of these houses lived a young man called Alban His father had sent him to school in Rome. After school he had served in the Roman army. Then he went back to his birthplace in Verulamuim.

The outcome   At the age of thirteen Henry no longer had any problems with reading or spelling and passed very rigorous exams to win a place at Westminster School, without any special allowance being made for his previous difficulties. He reads widely for pleasure now, and at the age of sixteen has already passed his first public examinations, called 'O levels' in Britain, in English Literature, English Grammar, French, History and Mathematics. At the time of writing, he is studying for his pre-university public examinations, or 'A levels', in History of Art, Early Medieval History and German. The predictions of his WISC test have turned out to be accurate: Henry is indeed better at the arts than sciences – proving that not all dyslexics are destined to become scientists, engineers or mechanics, as is popularly believed.

Henry's remarkable recovery shows not only that children who have early speech and language problems are not destined to do less well than other dyslexics, but also how early detection and treatment can place a child quickly back on an equal footing with his peers on the educational ladder. If Henry had been left to flounder until he was nine, ten, eleven or twelve, the chances of his catching up would not have been so good. By then he might have lost much of his self-confidence and interest in academic achievement, which helped to pull him through.

Cause for hope

Of all the children who were treated during my years at the St Bartholomew's Hospital Dyslexia Clinic, and who have been followed up, none is unemployed. They are now in their late teens or early twenties, and are either in further education or doing a job.

Of course, I have lost touch with some of them, but those with whom I have kept in contact all seem to be doing remarkably well. This is doubly encouraging if you take into account today's rising unemployment and educational cut backs. There are, I believe, three main reasons for their success.

1. I make no apology for repeating that recognition and treatment of dyslexia are vital – and the earlier the better. We cannot turn the clock back to see if Denis, Thomas, Janice and Henry would have become semi-literate adults had recognition and treatment not happened, but in my opinion there is that possibility. In any case, they might not have achieved their full intellectual potential. I am sure they would have done equally well at any other centre where similar multisensory, phonetically structured methods are used.

2. Another lesson is the importance of finding a good, qualified specialist teacher – just anyone who is sympathetic and warm will not do. The specialist teacher who hopes to tackle this sort of challenge successfully must know exactly what he or she is doing and why, otherwise all the warmth and understanding in the world will be to no avail. If all teachers were taught at training college how to teach reading and spelling to dyslexic children, perhaps many of these problems would be solved or at least lessened.

3. What seems to lie at the core of dyslexics' ability to succeed is the character and determination they so often bring to bear on their difficulties. In some cases, it is true, the will and determination only emerge relatively late, especially in those who were picked up late like Denis, but once they realize there is a chance of conquering their dyslexia, their desire to make up for lost time spurs them on, even at the age of sixteen, seventeen, or later still.

   I am constantly amazed at the courage with which dyslexic children endure, adapt to and often overcome their disabilities. Given the necessary encouragement and help by parents and teachers they are extraordinarily resilient. Many of the children we treated at the clinic had additional handicaps as well as the dyslexia, some of which were very severe. To find such indomitable and mature spirits in the young is surely a lesson to us all.

Our remedies oft in ourselves do lie,
Which we ascribe to heaven.

All's Well That Ends Well
William Shakespeare

8. COPING WITH DYSLEXIA

Unfortunately, not every dyslexic has the natural ability or the skilled teaching available to enable him to overcome his condition as fully as some of the children in the previous chapter. Many will continue to struggle with reading and writing throughout their time at school, some eventually managing to pass exams and move on to further education, others leaving school without qualifications. Even today, I am afraid, it can happen that a dyslexic child leaves school illiterate. I am often asked by anxious parents of older dyslexic children, 'Is there anything my boy can do to give him a better chance with his exams?', 'Will his dyslexia prevent him getting a job?', or, 'What sort of career is most suitable for dyslexics?' In this chapter I shall be attempting to answer these questions, as well as to give practical advice which husbands and wives, or partners, and close family can pass on to adults who have never learnt to read and write.

Advice for dyslexic students

By 'student' I mean any young person, from teenager at school to university student. Ideally by this time most young people should have been diagnosed dyslexic and should either have a specially geared teaching routine at school or be receiving specialist dyslexia therapy. Once they have finished their course of therapy they may not need any more specialist help, although some students benefit from occasional refresher courses, especially before taking exams. Whatever the situation, it is very important that parents or the student himself ensures that his tutor knows that he is dyslexic. I shall address the following sections directly to students, but if their dyslexia prevents them from tackling this part of the book, it should not be difficult for parents to pass the information on.

Hints on taking notes
It can be hard to take comprehensible notes from lessons or lectures, especially as many teachers and lecturers talk at speed, giving you hardly any time for note taking, and often rub things off the board before you have had a chance to copy them down correctly. Don't be afraid to ask for things to be repeated or further explained, or for visual material to be left on the board for longer. Your non-dyslexic friends will thank you for

this, as it is a common teaching fault. There are other ways around the problem too:

● If you have a very good memory, listen hard, make just a few key jottings to jog your memory and then write up as much as you can remember in the evening, double-checking with a friend to make sure that you have not missed anything vital. This will not be a nuisance for him or her, as they may well be glad to have someone to discuss the subject with in order to fill in some of the points which they themselves may have missed.

● Take a tape recorder to lessons or lectures and record them. You may have to ask permission to do this, but it's unlikely that it will be refused. This method is time-consuming, though, as you will have to listen to the tape several times later on in order to note down the salient points. But it will help to make sure you have missed nothing important and fix the information in your mind.

● Ask a friend to take notes with a carbon paper between pages so that there is a copy for you. Again, you can discuss the notes and the lesson or lecture later, which will benefit both of you.

● If you are good at keyboard work, either you or your school or college might like to invest in a revolutionary new hand-held wordprocessor called a Microwriter. It is worked by one hand, using a five-finger keyboard, and the system can be learned faster than standard ten-finger typing. Most people can reach longhand speed with around twenty-four hours of practice. Being pocket-size, it is very handy for taking notes in lectures or writing essays, since you can edit what you have written as it appears on a little display screen. You will need to have access to an electronic typewriter with memory facility (many schools and colleges have one) in order to get typewritten copy later on from the information stored in the Microwriter's memory. The Microwriter can be plugged into a typewriter, which then automatically types out everything you have keyed in previously. A basic Microwriter unit costs about as much as a golfball (Selectric) typewriter.

Hints on getting information from books

Reading books on your exam subject will probably take longer for you than for your non-dyslexic friends, so it's a great help if you know how to extract the information you need without having to read a book from cover to cover. The technique I recommend is as follows:

1. Read the contents page.
2. Decide which chapters you need to read.
3. Read the summaries at the end of these chapters to see if they will give you all the information you require.
4. Use the index to find the essential facts within the text.
5. Write down the important points contained in the book on index file

112

cards. Fill in as many cards as necessary, numbering each card as you go.
6. Clip the cards together and file them according to the author's surname.
7. Add the full reference for the book on a separate sheet of paper that lists all the books contained in the file. The best way to give the book its reference is to include the author's name(s), the date, the title and finally the town it was published in and the publisher, thus:

Goodman, J.F., (1975) *The Life Cycle of the Centipede*, London: Longmans.

8. Keep a separate filing box for each subject.

If you follow this procedure you will save a lot of time both by reducing the amount of essential material that you will need to revise before an exam, and by having full references immediately to hand when writing essays.

Hints on essay writing

Improve your vocabulary   One of the best ways of improving the quality of your essay writing is to build up a good vocabulary of apt and learned words. To do this, I would advise you to keep a personal dictionary in which you enter any word that you have difficulty in reading or spelling, and which you think will be useful to you later on. A pocket-size, loose-leaf, thumb-indexed notebook is ideal for the purpose. You should take it with you wherever you go, so as not to miss the opportunity of entering a new word you come across by chance, and so you can revise through the words in it from time to time – at least once a week if you can. It is particularly important to note down any specialized words that are needed for each subject and to make sure that you can spell these correctly.

Improve your general vocabulary by learning one new sophisticated word each week and entering it in your personal dictionary. Use it appropriately in as many of your essays as possible so that it becomes familiar enough to use with confidence in exams.

To begin with, choose words that are not too difficult to spell but that are commonly misused by dyslexics and non-dyslexics alike. It will be a feather in your cap if you use them correctly in essays and exams. Take the words 'militate' and 'mitigate', for example – very easy to spell, but very commonly misused. The word 'militate' is related to the word 'militant', so means 'fighting against'. In context you could use it thus: 'The fact that you only answered three questions when you should have answered four will militate against your chances of obtaining a good mark.' 'Mitigate', on the other hand, means to lessen the severity of. For instance, 'mitigating circumstances' are circumstances which lessen the severity of a crime.

Don't forget, when reading, to make a note of words you don't understand. Look them up later in a dictionary and add these to your vocabulary notebook if you think they are likely to be useful to you in the future. You may find it laborious to look things up, but a dictionary is one of your most valuable tools. It will not only give you the spelling and meaning of a word, but also tell you how to pronounce it and use it in sentences. Get into the habit of using a thesaurus too (a reference book which lists words by meaning rather than spelling) – a good way of enlarging your vocabulary and finding words that are more apt for expressing what you want to say in your essays.

Connecting your thoughts on paper I have found that right up until adulthood many dyslexics do not realize how their essays and other written work can be improved by using suitable connective words. Although they are often able to string ideas and sentences together well verbally, they usually find it hard to expand their ideas on paper. This is due not only to a limited written vocabulary but also to not using enough connective words that would help their written work to flow. Most of the youngsters I teach know how to use 'and' and 'but', but no others. The result is that their essays are halting and seem to lack maturity and confidence.

Connective words can be used to join up ideas within a sentence as well as to link the sentences themselves. 'Not only . . . but also' are useful connectors within a sentence. Without them you might write, 'I had committed a crime. I had failed to provide myself with an alibi.' How much better it reads like this: 'Not only had I committed a crime, but also had failed to provide myself with an alibi.'

Here are three simple sentences that sound disjointed in isolation:

It started to rain. I had brought my umbrella. I was able to stay dry.

By adding two connecting words, 'however' and 'so', you could turn it into two sentences that read well:

It started to rain. However, I had brought my umbrella, so I was able to stay dry.

There are, of course, many other common connectors that you should aim to add to your repertoire, such as: 'Nevertheless', 'therefore', 'indeed', 'thus', 'although', 'if', 'as', 'because', 'as well as', and so on.

The best way to start improving your use of connectors is to familiarize yourself with how they are used both in everyday speech and in the books, newspapers and magazines you read, and then practise including them in your essays and other written work. You will be surprised at the difference they will make.

114

Avoiding ambiguity   Dyslexics tend to put things in the wrong order when writing sentences, with the result that the ideas they are expressing relate to the wrong subject. This, coupled with the use of inappropriate words, often leads to ambiguity. In your essays try to make sure the reader will know exactly what you mean and that you have not altered your intended meaning by incorrect word or phrase order. The following example comes from one of my student's essays:

Cheap rail tickets should be used by elderly people before they expire.

This sounds as if the elderly should use their tickets before they die. By altering the wording and the order of the sentence, the meaning becomes unmistakeable.

Elderly people should use their cheap rail tickets before the expiry date.

Improving presentation   If your handwriting is bad – or even if it is not – a typewritten essay is much more professional looking than handwritten work, and is easier for your teacher or tutor to read. As long as your essay can be written out of class and you have your teacher's permission, if necessary, then it is definitely worth thinking about presenting your essays typewritten.

Although good typewriters are expensive, they will last a lifetime if properly looked after and can be a particularly good investment for the dyslexic. In my experience it is rare for dyslexics to find typing difficult, but if you want to type fast enough to make it worth while, you should learn to 'touch type', that is, to type without looking at the keys. There are many good teach-yourself books available, or you could take a short course of evening classes in your area.

Typing is a valuable skill for the dyslexic that will never be wasted. It will improve the presentation of your essays, your letters and, in fact, anything you write, making everything much neater and clearer. To avoid too many mistakes when typing, it helps to say each letter as you tap the keys – either aloud or in your mind – and to keep a steady rhythm rather than to be constantly speeding up and slowing down.

General essay-writing technique   Good essay writing is often the key to success at school, college or university. Marks for essays may have a big effect on your position in class, and many further education courses are based on continuous assessment of essay work. And of course in many subjects the essay may be the main form of answering questions in examinations.

If possible, always write your essays out in rough first (except in examinations, when time is at a premium), as it is much easier to think when writing in longhand, not having to worry about spelling. When you have finished your first draft, polish up the text with the aid of a dictionary and thesaurus. Double-checking everything should be second nature by now if you have had specialist remedial help. And you must adopt a really critical attitude to your written work to make sure that you have said exactly what you intended to say. Try also to look at your essay with a fresh eye, from a reader's point of view – this will help you to pick up any ambiguity that may have crept in. Finally, remember that constant essay-writing practice and noting how English is written by good authors will inevitably improve your style.

Hints on taking exams

Getting allowances made In most Western countries dyslexics can get allowances made for them in exams. In Britain you need a certificate, normally given by the psychologist who originally diagnosed you as dyslexic. Your school should arrange for you to have an up-to-date assessment for the certificate within eighteen months of sitting the exams. The head teacher or principal of your school or college will then send the certificate to the appropriate examining board. Most British examination boards accept certificates for dyslexics, allowing them extra time, or concessions for spelling – except, of course, for English. This is understandable, as spelling, grammar and sentence structure are what an English exam is all about. Remember, though, that many set, or required, books for English literature courses are available on tape. It may be possible to obtain extra time even for English. Severely dyslexic students should be able to obtain an amanuensis – someone to write down the answers which the dyslexic dictates – and, if necessary, a reader to read out the questions.

Before deciding exactly which exam you want to sit, it is worth taking the trouble to find out from the different examination boards the form the exams are likely to take. In other words, check whether questions require written answers or are set in a multiple-choice format. Multiple choice is obviously much easier for the dyslexic.

In some states in Australia, concessions, such as additional time, an amaneuensis, and use of a typewriter and thesaurus, are granted to dyslexic candidates for reference tests in English and mathematics. Also, if parents persist with their family doctor, their child's head teacher and school counsellor, it is possible to gain additional assistance in external exams.

In the United States, dyslexics wishing to take the high-school equivalency exam can obtain special editions of the exam, and special allowances, such as additional time, through the General Educational Development Testing Service (contact the Adult Education Agency in your state for details). American dyslexics may also obtain special allowances and/or editions of either of the two most commonly used college admissions/ placement tests – the Scholastic Aptitude Test (SAT) and the American College Testing (ACT) Assessment (for complete details, contact the appropriate oraganizations in the Appendix).

In Canada there is a growing awareness of the problems dyslexics face

116

in exams and increasing willingness to accommodate students whether by allowing extra time, putting the exam on tape or giving it orally.

Exam technique The following advice applies to anyone who will be sitting exams, but is doubly important for dyslexics. If you are worried that your lack of speed will prevent you finishing the paper – even if allowances are being made for time – you may tend to rush into the exam without taking enough time to check the questions.

1. Do not rush to begin writing the moment you are instructed to turn over the examination paper. First take a few calm deep breaths.
2. Read through the paper slowly and carefully, making sure you have understood what is required. When you are nervous it is all too easy to misread the questions and instructions. Double-check which questions are compulsory and which are optional. And most important of all, make absolutely sure how many questions you must answer in total. Decide which ones you are going to choose from the optional questions, and work out how long you can afford to spend on each question. Then start writing, beginning with a compulsory question.
3. Don't waste time making extensive notes first, as this takes up too many of the minutes you have allowed for that particular question. However, it is worth considering a simple plan first – perhaps list six simple headings so you have a basic structure to work to. As the theme develops while you are writing, other important points will occur to you. Jot these down immediately on a spare sheet of paper, otherwise, when you reach the point in your answer when you need to bring them in, you will have forgotten what they were.
4. Don't spend more than the time you have allotted yourself on any one question. If you only manage to answer three questions from a four-question paper you will automatically lose 25 per cent of your marks. This handicap can seldom be made up.
5. Give yourself ten minutes at the end, if you possibly can, to check your work over for spelling mistakes and left-out words. However, if you are still writing furiously when the examination comes to a close don't worry – chances are that you have done pretty well.

Careers for dyslexics

It's a widely held misconception that all dyslexics are unsuited to any job that requires reading and writing skills. This is not necessarily so. Provided that your condition has been recognized while you were young enough, and you have had suitable treatment, there is no reason why, by the time you start looking for a job, your initial handicap should not have been sufficiently overcome for you to make a success of any career you choose.

But you may think that however much your reading and writing skills have improved, you should definitely steer clear of such professions as doctor, nurse or pharmacist, because their mistakes with the written word can be life-threatening. Paradoxically, dyslexics who have made a career in medicine – and there are many – are probably less likely to make errors than their colleagues. One severely dyslexic friend of mine, a surgeon, had a very tough time at school, but managed to struggle through his medical exams, eventually to become one of Britain's leading brain surgeons. Although he now relies heavily on his secretary to handle the bulk of his written work, he has a nearly faultless record of writing out prescriptions – particularly where the dosage is concerned – because since childhood he has been in the habit of carefully double-checking everything he writes down.

There are different degrees of dyslexia, of course, and those whose reading and writing are very severely affected and who have not received adequate treatment would be wise not to choose to follow a career where mastery of these skills is a prime necessity – secretarial work and teaching English, for example. If your dyslexia is not severe, though, or has been improved by remedial teaching, then, in my view, provided you have the necessary ability, there is absolutely no career that is closed to you. I know successful dyslexic lawyers, academics, politicians, accountants, business executives and secretaries who cope with their disability by making good use of a dictionary and other people's help, and by taking extra care with their written work.

There is an encouraging study carried out in Maryland in 1968 by the sociologist, Prof Margaret Rawson, into the careers followed by dyslexic boys which shows that 14 per cent became research scientists, 13 per cent became business executives, 11 per cent became college professors, 7 per cent qualified as schoolteachers, 7 per cent as lawyers, and a further 7 per cent eventually owned or managed a business. These results cannot be taken as typical for all dyslexics because most of the boys' fathers were qualified professionals, and so family background clearly played a large part in the high proportion of success stories. However, this survey does show that dyslexics undoubtedly can succeed in areas where their disability is popularly thought to disqualify them.

Are there any jobs particularly suited to dyslexics?
While I don't want to give the impression that dyslexics only have a realistic chance of getting a job in certain fields, it does seem that certain innate abilities make a large proportion of dyslexics especially suited to particular types of work.

You may recall that in Chapter 3 I pointed out that many dyslexics have exceptional spatial ability, in other words are dextrous at two- and three-dimensional tasks which require visual skill. There are many jobs for which it is a distinct advantage to have good spatial ability, but perhaps there are

118

none as important in today's changing economic scene as computer operating and programming. (Remember, though, that dyslexics who don't have good spatial ability usually have poor visual and manual skills, but good language skills in spite of bad spelling – hence the many famous authors who have had dyslexic problems.)

Computers Although the arrival of microelectronic automation has contributed initially to raising the number of people out of work, it is a blessing in disguise for dyslexics. Take accounting, for example. In the past you needed crystal-clear handwriting to enter up figures in a ledger; now it can be largely a matter of punching keys. This opens up a whole new range of opportunities for dyslexics that was previously denied them. There is no doubt now that microelectronics is the industry of the future, and most dyslexics are particularly well equipped to take advantage of this. Their persistence, accuracy and speed at visual tasks such as keyboard work makes them ideal candidates for positions as trainee computer operators or programmers. It is true that many dyslexics have problems with the sequencing of everyday language, but they cope well with computer language, which is much more logical and regularly structured than the language we speak. Significantly, many of the programmers I have met seem to be dyslexic to some degree.

Dyslexic children often show a flair for operating home computers. Investing in a micro may help to prepare your child for his future profession.

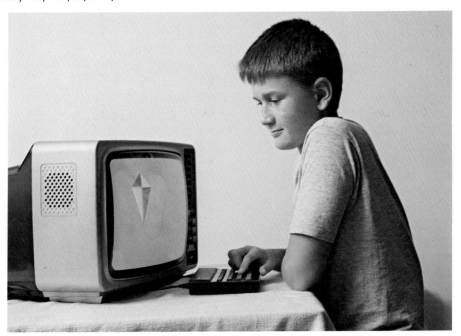

With home microcomputers now costing as little as the equivalent you would have to pay for a good transistor radio, parents can help to develop their children's interest in computers from the age of thirteen or earlier. A microcomputer at home gives a dyslexic youngster a new dimension in communication which he can really excel at, while giving him valuable experience that may well help to get him started in a career with a secure future. There is a wide range of computer software programs to help both children and adults with their literacy skills.

Other suitable jobs   There are scores of other jobs requiring a high level of spatial ability that suit a wide range of interests and intellectual levels. It would be impossible to mention them all, but the ones included in the following list are some of the most common.

Some jobs, careers and occupations requiring good spatial ability

- Advertising
- Agriculture/farming
- Ambulance service
- Architect
- Armed services (the military)
- Artist
- Bricklayer
- Builder
- Cameraman
- Car mechanic
- Carpenter
- Caterer
- Computer programmer/operator
- Construction work
- Craftsman
- Dancer
- Decorator
- Dentist
- Designer (graphic, fashion, industrial, interior, stage)
- Doctor
- Draughtsman
- Dressmaking
- Driver (bus, train, truck)
- Electrician
- Engineer
- Factory worker
- Fire service
- Forestry
- Gardener (landscape, market, nurseryman)
- Hairdresser
- Mechanic
- Merchant navy
- Musician
- Nurse
- Optician
- Osteopath
- Painter
- Petroleum exploration
- Photographer
- Physiotherapist
- Plumber
- Police
- Printing
- Reprographics
- Scientist
- Shop assistant
- Sports
- Surgeon
- Surveying
- Veterinary surgeon
- Welder

Dyslexics may also be good at jobs that rely heavily on verbal skill, since their difficulty in getting their thoughts down on paper does not usually extend to the spoken word. Quite the contrary in fact: many of my dyslexic pupils have been excellent talkers, as if to compensate for their lack of literary ability.

Some jobs and occupations requiring good verbal ability

- Barrister
- Businessperson
- Childcare
- Community worker
- Industrial relations work
- Lawyer
- Lecturer
- Marketing
- Personnel work
- Receptionist
- Salesperson
- Shop assistant
- Social worker
- Trade union official
- Travel courier/guide
- Politician

Hints on getting a job

● Go on any training courses that are relevant to the job. Many job training courses do not require you to have any previous qualifications and often run pre-course training in literacy and numeracy.

● Ask a friend or a member of your family to check over your application letter or form. Competition for jobs is so fierce nowadays that spelling mistakes or bad grammar can seriously jeopardize your chances of getting an interview. Applications stand a better chance of success if they are neatly typed out.

● Be confident at your interview. This is where dyslexics have their chance to shine, as most are articulate and can show their intelligence verbally.

● When going for an interview, first make an extra effort to dress smartly. Also, make sure you know exactly where you have to go, and that you are on time. These dyslexic problem areas are usually just a minor inconvenience, but could cost you a job at an interview.

● Don't mention that you are dyslexic, unless you have to. Although in practice your condition may make no difference to your ability to carry out the job properly, your prospective employer may not be well informed about dyslexia, and think that it is a sign of low intelligence. Don't lie about it, though. If you mention at your interview that you are dyslexic, explain that it is not related to intelligence and that it need not interfere with your work, as it is second nature for you to be extra careful with all your written work.

Hints for the young dyslexic at work

● Admit to your colleagues that you have difficulty with reading and writing. But instead of saying, 'I'm dyslexic', make a joke out of it: 'I'm

121

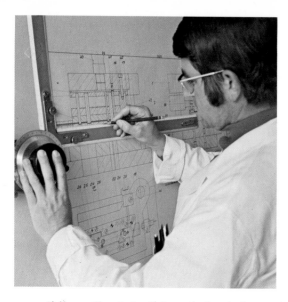

Most dyslexics have above-average spatial ability, which makes them ideally suited to careers in technical drawing and design.

a terrible speller.' And do ask for help with spelling. You will find most people will be very sympathetic – and many of your colleagues will be bad spellers themselves!

● Be especially careful when taking down telephone messages. Read back any numbers to check you have got them down correctly, and don't be afraid to ask the caller to repeat parts of the message (see also pages 124–5).

● Finally, and most important, don't let yourself be weighed down with anxiety and guilt about your dyslexia. This will cause you to lose confidence in yourself and in this way will be more harmful to your competence at your job than the dyslexia itself. Try to see its positive side. The determination and meticulous attitude you have had to develop since childhood to cope with your dyslexia will stand you in good stead when it comes to dealing with problems at work and holding down a job.

How adults can cope with dyslexia

As we have seen in the opening chapter, a surprisingly high proportion of adults are either semi-literate or completely illiterate – around two to three million in Britain out of a total population of nearly sixty million. And many more are probably dyslexic to a lesser degree. While in the United States there are estimated to be 23 million illiterate adults. As the vast majority of adults with reading and writing difficulties have never been professionally assessed, nobody knows how many are dyslexic, how many lacked sufficient education or how many simply don't have the intelligence to enable them to read and write. My guess is that many are dyslexic. Whatever the cause, the day-to-day problems are similar for all.

Despite not having benefited from current knowledge and remedial care during their formative years, most dyslexic adults manage to sort out their situation for themselves by developing their own strategies for coping with poor literacy. Although we live in a literate society, in some ways reading is not quite so important as it used to be, because radio and television provide a wealth of information which can be picked up without the ability to read. There are, though, several routine aspects of modern life where inability to read and write can be particularly problematic. Of course, a partner, family or close friends can help to make life a lot easier, but there are times when the adult needs to be equipped with the right techniques to be able to cope on his own. As previously in this chapter, I shall be addressing myself directly to the adult dyslexic, assuming that nearest and dearest will be passing on the advice.

Reading public signs

Fortunately many lettered public signs have been replaced by symbols or graphic signs – not, incidentally, to help the non-reader, but by international agreement to help foreign travellers who don't speak the language. GENTS and LADIES, which often caused embarrassment and confusion ten years ago have now by and large been superseded by graphic man and woman designs. However, there are a number of standard public signs that still need to be read, such as: IN, OUT, ENTRANCE, EXIT, EMERGENCY EXIT, FIRE DOOR, PUSH, PULL, BAR, RESTAURANT, TOILETS, WC, PARKING, PUBLIC, PRIVATE, PAY HERE, STOP, GO, WALK, SLOW, CAUTION, DANGER, POLICE, FIRST AID, KEEP OFF THE GRASS, and so on. These, or at least the really important ones like DANGER and EXIT, should be memorized by sight. The best way to do this is to get someone to write down the wording for each sign in capital letters on a card. Then practice with that person matching the signs on the cards to the word spoken aloud until the meaning has become clear and the word imprinted on your memory.

If you are travelling to a train, underground or subway station you do not know, make sure that you either check with someone before leaving home on the number of stations you have to pass before arriving at the stop you want, or ask one of the railway staff, or fellow passengers.

Labels and instructions

Not being able to read instructions can lead to disaster. There have been cases where adults with a heart condition have died because they were not able to read the instructions on pill bottles explaining how to open child-proof tops. Obviously, it is vital that partners or family should explain and clarify all the instructions and labels relating to dangerous or life-saving items in the house. For example, the dyslexic adult must be kept fully informed about drugs in the family medicine cupboard; poisonous chemicals that are used around the house, in the garden or for amateur photography; as well as about the instructions for using a fire extinguisher and the colour coding for electrical wiring, which is occasionally subject to change.

Driving
Some dyslexics are very bad at judging speed and distances, so will not be able to drive a car, most, though, are no more likely to fail the driving test than those who can read normally. Nearly all road signs consist of symbols or designs rather than letters, and the Highway Code can be learnt by heart if someone puts it on tape for you.

Following maps or directions can be a nightmare, though, especially if you have directional confusion as well, so that you are not sure which is left and right, north and south, east and west. If you can't arrange for someone else to navigate for you, ask for directions to be given relating to landmarks, like this: 'Turn away from the bridge when you get to the junction', instead of: 'Turn left when you get to the junction.' You might find it helpful to memorize whether the hand you write with is left or right, and then to mark the back of that hand clearly in washable ink for the duration of the journey. Or you could mark an 'R' and an 'L' on the car windscreen.

Filling in forms
If your dyslexia is severe, there is no way round form filling other than asking either someone at home or an official to do it for you. There is no need to feel reticent about asking for professional assistance – they are used to helping out, as few people really understand official forms anyway!

Telephone messages
The biggest worry I have found among severely dyslexic adults is fear of being expected to take down telephone messages. There are three ways of approaching this problem.

1. Arrange to have your telephone linked up with a tape recorder to which the message can be transmitted.
2. Explain to the person who is giving the message that you are a terrible speller and ask him or her to spell out their message, name and telephone number carefully and slowly.
3. If the message is too long and complicated, take down the caller's details, and explain that you are unable to take down the message and will ask the person the caller is trying to reach to ring back.

An added difficulty for the dyslexic when taking down messages is that the telephone only handles a limited sound frequency range, so certain sounds are easily distorted and confused. The sound /b/ often resembles /v/ and vice versa; and the letters 'f', 's' and 'c' are often nearly impossible to tell apart when people are spelling them out over the telephone. To avoid mistakes, most people use a code for identifying the letters: ' "C" for Charlie', ' "S" for sugar', ' "F" for Freddie' and so forth. Unless care is taken, the code itself can muddle a dyslexic – if the first letter-sound of the code word does not precisely match the letter it is meant to represent. This is the case with the three examples used above, the sound /ch/ in 'Charlie' being paired with 'C', the sound /sh/ in 'sugar' with 'S', and the blend /fr/ in Freddie with the letter 'F'. The dyslexic should invent his own system where the first letter of the code word sounds exactly like the alphabet letter it is being paired with – ' "C" for carrot', ' "S" for signal', ' "F" for fig', for example.

The way ahead

Many severely dyslexic adults will be able to rely on their partners, family and perhaps secretaries to do most of the reading and writing for them. The trouble is that the less you use a skill, the rustier it becomes. So the best advice is to press on alone and struggle with it whenever you can.

It is worth remembering that, in Britain at least, dyslexia is now legally recognized as a handicap within the official group of 'Specific Learning Difficulties'. If you are a registered dyslexic, and your condition is severe enough, you will qualify as a handicapped person, a number of whom have to be included on the payrolls of companies over a certain size. Of course, to be registered as dyslexic you will need to have been diagnosed. So if your disability was not checked when you were younger, you should arrange to have an assessment with a psychologist – either approaching one direct, or via your family doctor if you rely on a public health scheme.

If you feel that your lack of reading and writing skills is completely disrupting your life, then perhaps you should consider applying to join a course at a dyslexia teaching centre, as most cater for adults as well as children (see Appendix for addresses). Or if there isn't a centre near you you might try an adult literacy course organized by a local further education college or by adult community education. Ask at your public library or local education authority for details.

Happily, not all adult dyslexics are completely illiterate. Many learn to read well enough to get by, even if writing remains very difficult. Still, postal letters are not the only means of communication; there is always the telephone, or you can use a miniature tape recorder, or dictaphone, to dictate letters onto for transcription or typing later, or you can send a tape direct to someone who has a compatible tape recorder. In any case there is no shame in being dyslexic – some of the world's most brilliant people have been atrocious readers and spellers (see pages 10–12). But you will need to learn to accept and live with your dyslexia, and to anticipate the problems that are likely to occur so that you can improvise your way around them.

9. DYSLEXIA AND THE BRAIN

Some of the ideas in this chapter are rather more complicated than those in the rest of this book. But I hope they will be of interest to parents and teachers of dyslexics, as they help to explain many of the points covered in previous chapters and to clarify to some extent the underlying causes of dyslexia. It is perfectly possible, though, to understand and benefit from the other chapters in the book without reading this one.

It is now becoming widely accepted by specialists that a dyslexic's brain cells are arranged differently to a greater or lesser degree from a normal reader's. Since you inherit your brain cell arrangement in much the same way as you inherit aspects of your personality and your physical characteristics, it is not surprising that 88 per cent of dyslexics have close family with the condition. Although, as I have mentioned before, some people's dyslexia is caused by changes in the brain resulting from illness or accident, normally before, during or just after birth. Whether hereditary or not, the extent of the difference in brain cell arrangement determines whether someone's dyslexia is mild, moderate or severe.

Language and the two hemispheres

We still do not understand exactly how the brain works, but we are fairly sure of what happens in its various areas. Each area has a different function but reacts with others around it, enabling the brain to work as an interrelating whole. The brain is split into two separate halves – a right and a left hemisphere – which can communicate with each other by a 4-in (10-cm) long connecting set of nerve fibres called the corpus callosum (see diagram opposite). Although the two hemispheres look the same, they usually perform very different tasks. In broad terms, for most people the left side is the verbal, logical and controlling half, while the right is the non-verbal, practical, intuitive side.

In most people's brains, language is processed mainly in the left hemisphere. Broca's area (see diagram on page 128) is involved in the mechanics of expressing language, and Wernicke's area is where our understanding of speech takes place. As you can see from the diagram, people also have a language area in their right hemisphere, which is smaller and much less efficient in processing and organizing language-based skills.

Most of the research into where language is processed in the brain has been conducted on persons who have had strokes or accidents of some kind. Usually such patients are middle-aged or elderly, so age-related changes tend to interact with the underlying damage. In 1967 Prof Oliver Zangwill of Cambridge University found that 98 per cent of right-handers experienced severe speech difficulties after damage to the left side of the brain, whereas speech was affected in less than 2 per cent of right-handers whose right hemispheres were damaged. The picture is less clear with left-handers who may have language more evenly distributed between the two hemispheres.

More precise information was obtained in 1973 by Prof Alexander Romanovich Luria, the eminent Soviet neuropsychologist at Moscow University. He studied war victims who had sustained penetrating head wounds and observed what they could no longer do. As it was possible to ascertain exactly where the fragment had entered the brain and the patients were young and had previously intact cerebral function, the results of the research were more reliable. Although there is still some uncertainty, approximately 95 per cent of right-handers are considered to have language sited in their left, or dominant hemispheres.

Many specialists now believe that dyslexic difficulties could arise when someone's language areas are split more evenly between the two halves of the brain. The source of the problem seems to lie in the connection between

The corpus callosum links the two halves of the brain. The anterior commissure is a smaller link. If the former is severed, the two halves work independently.

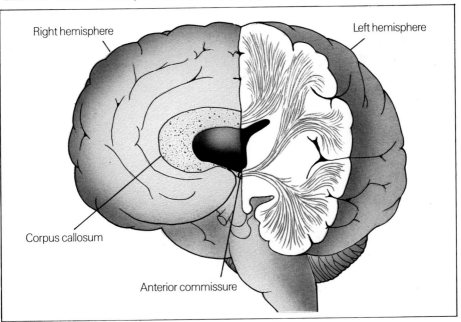

Right hemisphere

Left hemisphere

Corpus callosum

Anterior commissure

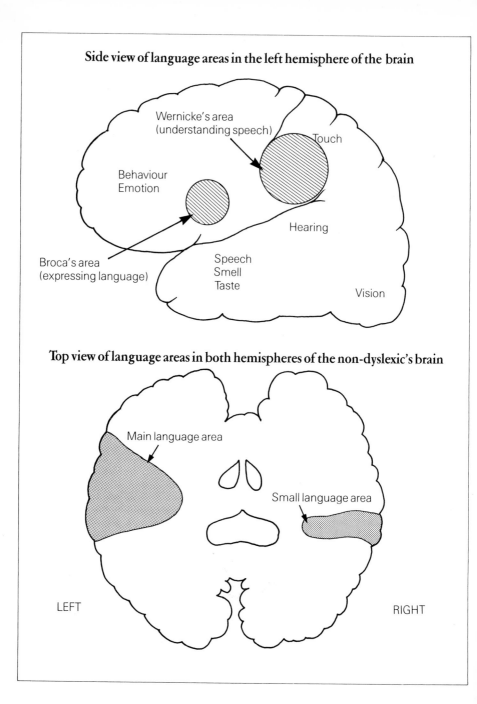

Side view of language areas in the left hemisphere of the brain

Wernicke's area
(understanding speech)

Touch

Behaviour
Emotion

Broca's area
(expressing language)

Speech
Smell
Taste

Hearing

Vision

Top view of language areas in both hemispheres of the non-dyslexic's brain

Main language area

Small language area

LEFT

RIGHT

Two views of the non-dyslexic brain. ABOVE: The main language areas are situated in the left half of the brain. BELOW: There are language areas in both halves of the brain, although the one on the right is much smaller.

the two hemispheres – the collection of nerve fibres called the corpus callosum. In 1974 Prof Tim Miles of Bangor University in north Wales carried out research into how quickly dyslexics' brains process the information received from visual symbols. Volunteers were asked to watch numbers flash rapidly in front of them on a machine called a tachistoscope. Even dyslexic university students perceived them slower and less accurately than nine-year-old non-dyslexics, and the non-dyslexics also managed to retain sequences in the memory better. This suggests that in the dyslexics' brains more messages had to be passed from one hemisphere to the other for the numbers to be identified and named. It is as if a confusing traffic jam of nerve signals builds up in the corpus callosum between the language areas in the opposite sides of the brain, complicating a dyslexic's understanding and expression of verbal or written speech.

In line with this theory, recent anatomical research in 1981 by Dr Albert Galaburda and Dr Thomas Kemper from Boston in the United States has brought to light noticeable anatomical differences between dyslexics' and normal readers' brains. Investigating the brain of a dyslexic who died in his twenties, they found unusual arrangements of cells which suggested that the language areas were distributed more equally than usual on either side of the brain.

Before the brain can interpret language, it has to perceive the written and spoken word. And so we turn now to the way in which sight and hearing react with the brain.

Perception and understanding of sight and sound

Vision

I do not want to go into every complexity of the routes taken by visual impulses from the eye along the nervous pathway to the brain, because they are not essential to the understanding of dyslexia and will only be confusing. Broadly speaking, though, each eye has its own field of vision, and when you look straight at an object close to you, it falls within the overlap of the two fields of vision. So when the image of this single object falls on the retina at the back of the eye, it sets up nerve impulses from both eyes which arrive at the visual cortices – areas at the back of both hemispheres of the brain, where the image is actually perceived (see diagram overleaf). To complicate matters, the image that falls on to the retina is upside down and back to front. It is up to the brain to interpret the nerve signals from this image so that we perceive the object as it really is, the right way round and the right way up.

The brain does not have much trouble in analysing the shape of solid objects such as a chair, because from whichever angle it is viewed, it can

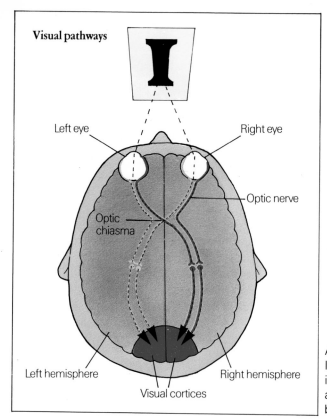

Visual pathways

Left eye

Right eye

Optic nerve

Optic chiasma

Left hemisphere

Right hemisphere

Visual cortices

A diagram showing how a letter sets up visual impulses that are received at the visual cortices in both halves of the brain.

only be a chair. Analysing abstract symbols like letters and numbers is more difficult because by switching the same shape around you can get different letters and numbers. The 'b' shape, for example, turns into 'd' when turned back to front, becomes 'q' if you turn 'd' upside down, and 'p' if you then flip 'q' back to front – four letters from one shape. So, if you were asked to pick out the letter 'p' from:

b   d   p   q

your brain would have to be able to recognize the correct image and reject the incorrect ones. To do this the visual impulses received in the visual cortices at the back of both hemispheres have to be analysed by the logical language area of the brain. If you have your language area on the left side, as it usually is, then it is likely that only one set of messages is transmitted for interpretation across the corpus callosum from the right-hand visual cortex to the analytical language area in the left hemisphere. Whereas if you have substantial language areas in both the right and the left hemispheres – as it seems many dyslexics do – then the corpus callosum, which joins up the hemispheres, will get clogged up with a mass of interconnecting signals

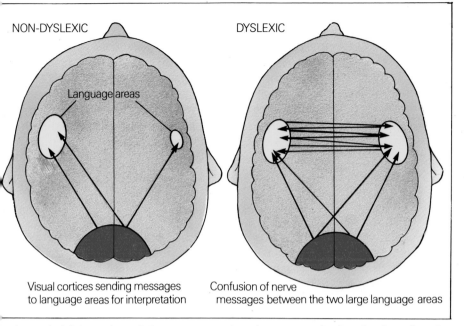

Language areas

Visual cortices sending messages
to language areas for interpretation

Confusion of nerve
messages between the two large language areas

A theoretical impression of the way nerve impulses set up in the visual cortices by seeing a letter might travel for interpretation to the language areas of the brain. In the dyslexic (right) the corpus callosum would become 'jammed' with nerve impulses as the two large language areas refer the messages they are receiving from the visual cortices back and forth for comparison and analysis.

between visual cortices and language areas in both hemispheres (see diagram above). This confusion of nerve messages may be why dyslexics often read 'b's as 'd's and vice versa.

In addition to this problem, Dr George Pavlidis, currently working in the United States, discovered in 1979 that when dyslexics read, they make larger, jerkier eye movements than normal readers do. This may partly account for the way dyslexics tend to reverse word and letter order when reading.

Convergence As I mentioned in Chapter 6, if our eyes cannot converge together properly to look at an object, this makes it difficult to make sense of the letters and words that are being read.

When the muscles controlling the eyes point the pupils directly at a letter, its image – which is slightly different in each eye – falls on matching points in the two retinas. When the images hit the right places in the retinas, the two sets of nerve signals are fused by the visual cortex so that only one letter is seen.

When convergence is not correct, the images of the letter will hit points of the retinas which do not match. The two sets of nerve messages cannot therefore be fused by the visual cortex and two letters will be seen when you are really only looking at one. Most people with this problem learn to accept one image and reject the other. Some, though, do not develop a fixed reference eye for reading and therefore continue to see either two images or to switch from one image to the other. This, of course, makes reading extremely difficult. Around 30 per cent of children with reading difficulties do not have a fixed reference eye. You can get an idea of the problem they have by closing one eye and looking at one word on this page; now open that eye, simultaneously closing the other one and keeping your attention on the same word. It will appear to jump across the page. If you don't have a fixed reference eye, this is the sort of visual trick that can plague your reading.

Current research shows that dyslexic children who have been found to have no firmly established reference eye for reading have been helped to develop one under expert supervision by patching of the left eye. Originally, if the dyslexic was left-handed, the right eye was patched to avoid him becoming a crossed lateral – left-handed and right-eyed (see page 81) – and vice versa if he was right-handed. Nowadays the left eye is patched for reading and writing, regardless of handedness, to encourage right-eye-to-left-hemisphere processing of written language – the left side of the brain being, of course, the better for this type of activity. Research into the effects of eye patching is still in progress, so it must only be used under professional guidance and cannot yet be practised as a self-help technique.

Hearing

Not only do dyslexics muddle up the shape and order of the letters and words they see, but also tend to confuse the order of syllables and numbers which they hear spoken aloud. Although this can be due to hearing loss resulting from something wrong with the ear itself, it is more often due to the way the brain interprets the nerve impulses sent by the ears. If there is the slightest hitch at any point in the hearing process – from the point where sound waves enter the ear to the moment they are understood in the brain – perception of speech may become confused.

The deciphering of speech sounds in the brain is an incredibly complex procedure. The brain has to analyse every single sound before it can be understood, and when you consider that, unlike with reading, you often have no control over the speed at which the sounds of speech bombard your hearing, it is remarkable that we pick up the skill at all, and not surprising that as with any elaborate piece of precision machinery there is so much scope for it to go wrong.

You can see from the diagram opposite that nerve impulses created by sound waves inside the ears travel along nerve fibres to areas called the auditory cortex in both hemispheres of the brain. Although impulses from each ear go to both hemispheres, the nerve pathways which cross over are much stronger. Therefore sounds heard in the right ear are mostly interpreted in the left hemisphere and vice versa.

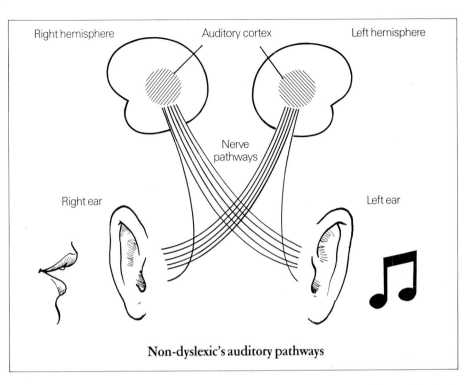

Non-dyslexic's auditory pathways

A theoretical impression of the way nerve impulses created by sounds travel to both halves of the brain from each ear. The crossed pathways are stronger, so what is heard in the right ear is mostly interpreted in the left hemisphere, and vice versa.

Once again, it seems as if the siting of the language areas in the dyslexic's brain plays a crucial part in his ability to decipher the spoken word. In non-dyslexics the right ear tends to be better at interpreting speech sounds because of its stronger connection with the language area in the left-hand side of the brain. And the left-ear-to-right-hemisphere connection is better at making sense of non-verbal noises like slamming doors, dripping taps and music. So-called 'dichotic listening tests', in which different sets of spoken words or numbers are played at the same speed and volume into different earpieces in a set of headphones (see page 86), show that many severe dyslexics either prefer to interpret the speech sounds coming into their left ear, ignoring those played into the right ear, or show no particular preference for listening to verbal material with either ear. This suggests that their language areas are not mainly in the left hemisphere. As we have seen, once the brain has to start analysing language in both hemispheres at once, the connection between the two halves through the corpus callosum may become overloaded, creating confusion in the dyslexic's mind about what he is trying to interpret.

Can these difficulties be overcome?

Faced with such fundamental problems, you could be forgiven for wondering how the dyslexic child can be expected to make any headway at all against his disability. Fortunately, though the cause of dyslexia seems to lie in the arrangement of cells in his brain, hope for recovery can be found in the young brain's ability to change and adapt to new stimuli.

All successful multisensory dyslexic teaching of the type described in Chapters 5 and 7 is based on an awareness of the complete cycle of nerve impulses that is involved in dyslexia. Suppose a child is shown a letter 'd', told what it is and then asked to copy it and say out loud what he has copied. First, his brain receives the visual and spoken information about the letter, then it decides what it might mean, sets the writing hand in motion to copy the letter, monitors the results of this action – both through the nerve signals fed back by the hand and arm muscles as they write and through the visual impulses created by the newly written letter, as well as through the auditory clue of reading aloud what has been written down. If the child is dyslexic, one or more parts of this cycle will not be working properly. Yet since his nervous system is programmed to make sense of the world, it will tend to impose an order of its own if a normal one is denied to it. So, for example, he may see the letter 'd', perceive it as a 'b', write it as a 'b' and confidently read it back as a 'd'. If teaching follows a similar circular pattern, so everything he sees and hears is first made comprehensible, then he is taught how to translate it into written form and then to read it back correctly, gradually the faulty links in his dyslexic cycle will be bridged.

A young child's brain cells are able to adapt and change, but this flexibility becomes less as the brain matures. It seems that there are two critical periods for acquiring language: from birth to five years for spoken language and up to fifteen for written language. Of course, this does not mean that you cannot learn anything new after you reach fifteen, but after that age the functions of the various different areas in the brain become fixed and lose their ability to change. Since the aim of dyslexic therapy is to alter the way in which the brain organizes and processes language, it is obvious why teaching should be started as soon as possible and why results with the older dyslexic are less good.

The young brain's ability to change often results in the dyslexic child ending up with certain advantages over his non-dyslexic friends. Because the type of remedial teaching just described is nearly always effective, the dyslexic need not be hampered by lack of literary skills. And as if to compensate for his original disabilities, his brain may well have endowed him with high-level talents in other fields such as mathematics, the sciences and creative activities such as painting, music or sculpture, in addition to providing him with an extra measure of persistence and determination. *Vive la difference!*

USEFUL ADDRESSES

UNITED KINGDOM
National

British Dyslexia Association
98 London Road
Reading
Berkshire RG1 5AU
Tel: (0734) 668271/2

College of Speech Therapists
Harold Poster House
6 Lechmere Road
London NW2 5BU

Dyslexia Association of Northern Ireland
39 High Street
Hollywood
County Down

National Library of Talking Books for the Handicapped
12 Lant Street
London SE1
Tel: 071 407 9417

Scottish Dyslexia Association
Cakemuir House
Nenthorn, Kelso
Roxburghshire
Tel: (0573) 24806

Teaching and assessment centres

Arkell Dyslexia Centres
Frensham
Farnham
Surrey GU10 3BW

Development Centre
Hide Place
Vincent Square
London SW1P 4JN

Dyslexia Institute
133 Gresham Road
Staines TW18 1SB

Dyslexia Teaching Centre
23 Kensington Square
London W8

Hampstead Dyslexia Clinic
78 Oakwood Road
London NW11

The Hornsby Centre
71 Wandsworth Common Westside
London SW18 2ED
Tel: 081 871 2691/1092

Knowle Hill Remedial Centre
Cherwell
Knowle Hill
Woking, Surrey

Universities

Dyslexia Unit
Department of Psychology
University of North Wales
Bangor LL57 2DG

Centre for the Teaching of Reading
University of Reading
Bulmershe Court
Earley, Reading RG6 1HY
Berkshire
Tel: (0734) 352742

Hospitals

Bloomfield Learning Centre
Guy's Hospital
London SE1

Dyslexia Clinic
West Wing
St Bartholomew's Hospital
London EC1A 7BE

Specialist Schools

Appleford School (junior)
Shrewton
Salisbury SP3 4HL
Wiltshire

Eastcourt School
Victoria Parade
Ramsgate
Kent

Edington School (junior)
Mark Road
Burtle, Near Bridgwater
Somerset TA7 8NJ

Fairly House
44 Bark House
London W2 4AT

Hornsby Hall (junior)
Kyrle Road
London SW11

Mark College (senior)
Mark House
Mark, Highbridge
Somerset TA9 4NP

Millfield School (senior)
Street
Somerset

The Old Rectory (junior)
Brettenham
Near Ipswich
Suffolk

Ravenscroft
Farleigh Castle
Near Bath
Avon

St David's College (senior)
Llandudno
Gwynedd
North Wales

Shapwick School (senior)
Burtle
Near Bridgwater
Somerset

Shiplake College (senior)
Henley-on-Thames
Oxfordshire RG9 4BW

Stanbridge Earls (senior)
Romsey
Hampshire SO5 0ZS

School with specialist unit

Hornsby House School (junior)
Broomwood Methodist Hall
Kyrle Road
London SW11 6JX

Educational Books

Ann Arbor Publishing Inc
PO Box 1
Belford
Northumberland NE70 7JX

Bath Educational Books Ltd
7 Walcot Buildings
London Road
Bath BA1 6AD

Heinemann Educational Books
Halley Court
Jordan Hill
Oxford OX2 8EJ

Souvenir Press
43 Great Russell Street
London WC1B 3PA

Teaching Materials

Alpha to Omega – the A-Z of teaching
    reading, writing and spelling
Bevé Hornsby and Frula Shear
Heinemann Educational

Alpha to Omega Flashcards
Bevé Hornsby
Heinemann

Alpha to Omega Activity Pack
Bevé Hornsby and Julie Pool
Heinemann Educational

Alpha to Omega Pelmanism Pairs Games
Bevé Hornsby and Catriona Fitzgerald
Hornsby Centre

Bangor Teaching Programme
Elaine Miles

Before Alpha
Bevé Hornsby, Souvenir Press

Help for Dyslexic Children
Tim Miles and Elaine Miles
Methuen

Move in Time – Exercises in Coordination
Mary Nash-Wortham
68 Pashley Road
Eastbourne

Practical Guide to Children's Handwriting
Rosemary Sassoon
Thames & Hudson

The Development of Handwriting Skills
Christopher Jarman
Basil Blackwell

Educational Equipment and Toys

James Galt & Co Ltd
30-31 Great Marlborough Street
London W1

LDA – Learning Development Aids
(also suppliers of educational software for
microcomputers)
Duke Street
Wisbech
Cambridgeshire PE13 2AE

AUSTRALIA
National

**Association for Children with Learning
Disabilities (ACLD)**
21-3 Belmore Street
Burwood 2134
New South Wales

**Australian Federation of SPELD Associations
(AUSPELD)**
c/o SPELD NSW
PO Box 94
16 Coronation Avenue
Mosman, New South Wales 2088

Local

SPELD ACT
PO Box 129
Kingston 2604

SPELD Queensland
27 McDougall Street
Milton 4064

SPELD South Australia
PO Box 83
Glenside 5065

SPELD Tasmania
PO Box 154, North Hobart 7002

SPELD Victoria
494 Brunswick Street
Fitzroy 3065

SPELD Western Australia
PO Box 61
Mosman Park 2604

BAHAMAS

The Bahamas Council for the Handicapped
PO Box N3938
Nassau

BAHRAIN

Dyslexic Support Group
(Mrs C. Hewitson)
c/o Reuters, PO Box 1426
Deira, Dubai
United Arab Emirates

BELGIUM

APEDA
(Presidente: Madame S. De Maerschalck)
12 Rue du Prinptemps
1328 Ohain

BERMUDA

The Reading Clinic
Cave House
Harbour Road
Warwick
Tel: 6-3302

BFPO

SO2 SCEA 1b
Director of Army Education
Ministry of Defence
Court Road
Eltham, London SE9 5NR

BRAZIL

Associacao Brasileira de Dyslexia (ABD)
(President: Roberto d'Utra Vaz)
Rua Sergipe 475
7 Angar, Sala 705
Sao Paulo

CANADA

**The Canadian Association for Children and
Adults with Learning Disabilities**
Maison Kildare House
323 Chapel Street
Suite 200
Ottawa KIN 7Z2
Tel: 613 238 5721
*This association has divisions across Canada in
each Province*

Edmonton Association for Children with SLD
Apartment 302
10010–105 Street
Edmonton, Alberta

Ontario Association for Children with SLD
1901 Yonge Street
Suite 504
Toronto, Ontario M4S 2Z3

Vancouver Branch of the Orton Dyslexia Association
(President: Mrs Anne Parsons)
Box 35322, Station E
Vancouver BC
V6M 4G5

The Reading Foundation
#250-200 Rivercrest Drive S.E.
Calgary AB T2C 2X5

CZECHOSLOVAKIA

Child Guidance Clinic
(Dr Joroslav Sturma)
Prague 9 25095
Dolni Pocernice

DENMARK

Landsforening For Orblindesagen I Denmark
Vejlesovij 41
DK 2840 Holte

FINLAND

Suomen Puhe-Luigyholistus Finra
Suomen Sonopedis-Foniatrinem Yhoistus
Her Kam Ruotto
Kielokatn 13
80130 Joensun

FRANCE

Union Nationale France Dyslexie
(President: Monsieur Jean-Francois Houlard)
4 Rue P. Guilbert, 91330 Yerres
Tel: 69 48 0899

(Secretariat: Madame M. Montarnal)
3 bis, avenue des Solitaires,
78320 Le Mesnil
Saint Denis
Tel: 16 (1) 34.61.96.43

GERMANY

Bundesverband Legasthenie, e.V.
(President: Dr Lisa Dummer)
Gneisenaustrasse 2
3000 Hanover I
Tel: 0511 853465

GREECE

Association for Parents of Children with Dyslexia
(Presidente: Madame Verychaki)
Saint Konstantin 6
Amonia, Athens

GUATEMALA

Secretario Ejecutivo de lOs Impedidos
14 Calle 0-28
Zona 3, Guatemala
Tel: 83566 83572

HONG KONG

SPELD Hong Kong
PO Box 95860, Tsim Sha Tsui, Kowloon

INDIA

Alpha to Omega Centre
1 Manikeswam Road
Kilpark, Madras 600010
India

Indian Dyslexia Association
Mistral, 331A Firtree Road
Epsom Downs, Surrey KT17 3LG
(Mrs Janice Kapoor)

ISRAEL

Dyslexia Association for Parents of Children with Dyslexia
(Mrs C. Rotstein)
Sharon Eshkoli 124/33
Ramot, Jerusalem

NITZPAN
5 Peretz Haiot Street
Tel Aviv 63262

Israel Association for Learning Disabled Children
School of Education
The Hebrew University
Jerusalem

ITALY

Mrs Wardle (forming an Association)
Via Talete 36
Rome

JAMAICA

**Jamaica Association for Children with
  Learning Disabilities**
(Administrator: Miss Maisie Reid)
c/o British High Commission
PO Box 575
Trafalgar Road
Kingston 10

KUWAIT

Center for Child Evaluation and Teaching
(General Manager: Faten Al-Bader)
PO Box 5433, Safat
Tel: 845221

MALTA

The Malta Dyslexia Association
(Rev Br. H.A. Clews)
St Benild's School
Sliema

NETHERLANDS

Stichting Dyslexie
Postbus 1558
6501 Nijmegen

De Pyler
Willebrordstraat 80
1970 A.C. Ijmuiden
Tel: 02550 30599

NEW ZEALAND

**New Zealand Federation of Specific Learning
  Difficulties Association Inc**
PO Box 28-119
Auckland

SPELD New Zealand
PO Box 13391
Christchurch

NORWAY

Norsk Dysleksiforbund
Sporvies gt. 10
Oslo 3

Specialskolen for Thalehemmed
Bredtvet
Oslo 9

PAKISTAN

Dyslexia Association of Pakistan
(Mr Shad Moarif)
D-208 Shalamar Estates
Clifton V
Karachi 6

PORTUGAL

St Julians School (forming an Association)
Susan Nures
Carcavelos
2777 Parede-Codex

PUERTO RICO

League to Aid Children with SLD
Universidad de Puerto Rico
PO Box 5067
San Juan 00946

SINGAPORE

Lorna Whiston Study Centre
35 Selegie Road
05-09 Parklane Shopping Mall
Singapore 0718
Tel: 3363969

SOUTH AFRICA

**The Association for Learning and
  Educational Difficulties**
44 Wolfgang Avenue
Norwood 2192
Johannesburg

Japari Remedial Education Centre
1 Dundalk Avenue
Parkview
Johannesburg

Rebecca Ostrowick School of Reading
(Edna Frenkel)
PO Box 4106, 5 Selkirk Street
Germston South 1401

**South African Association for Children with
  Learning and Educational Difficulties**
Division Specialised Education
University of Witwatersrand
1 Jan Smuts Drive
Johannesburg

SPAIN

Fundacio Centro de Estudios de Aprendizaje
y Reeducacion
Paseo de Moret 9
Madrid

Centre d'estudi i tractament de dislexia
Montserrat Estilles
Rios Rosas 5
08006 Barcelona

SWEDEN

Svenska Dyslexiforbundet
(President: Dr Britta Wassmouth)
Skleppstavagen 16, S-12430 Bandhagen
Stockholm SDF

Mrs S. Janerus
FMLS Moranvaden 4
19171 Sollentunn

SWITZERLAND

DELEGA
(President: Madam Liselotte Bacher)
Gruzefeldstrasse 40
8400 Winterthur

TRINIDAD

The Association for Developmental
Education
c/o La Jeunesse Tutorials
Corner Tragarete Road and Elizabeth Street
Port-of-Spain

Remedial Centre (1986)
9 Union Road
Marballa

UNITED STATES OF AMERICA

Information

American Speech, Language and Hearing
Association
10801 Rockville Pike
Rockville MD 20852

Association for Children with Learning
Disabilities
4156 Library Road
Pittsburgh, PA 15234

The Orton Dyslexia Society Inc
724 York Road
Baltimore
Maryland 21204
Tel: 301 296 0232

Californian Association for Neurologically
Handicapped Children
PO Box 1160
El Cerrito, CA 94530

Materials and remedial reading

Academic Therapy Publications
20 Commercial Boulevard
Novato, CA 94947

Ann Arbor Publishing Inc
PO Box 7249
Naples, FL 33940

Educator's Publishing Service Inc
75 Moulton Street
Cambridge, MA 02238

For information on special allowances in examinations

ACT Assessment – Special Testing Guide
Test Administration
PO Box 168, Iowa City
1A 52243

ATP: Services for Handicapped Students
Institutional Services
Box 592, Princeton NJ 08541

YUGOSLAVIA

SUVAG Anke Butorac 10, 41000 Zagreb

European Dyslexia Association

(Chairman: Marcel Seynave)
avenue Charles Woeste 38
Bt. 7-1090, Brussels
(Secretary: Anne-Marie Montarnal)
46 av. Port-Royal-des-Champs
78320 Le Mesnil Saint Denis, France

The British Dyslexic Association has contacts in many countries, so if there is a particular country not included on this list for which you require a contact, the Association Office may be able to give the name and address of someone who could help.

INDEX

Page numbers in *italic* refer to the illustrations.